Infertility and Adoption:
A Guide for
Social Work Practice

Infertility and Adoption: A Guide for Social Work Practice

Deborah Valentine
Editor

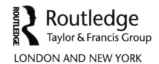

Routledge
Taylor & Francis Group

LONDON AND NEW YORK

First published 1988 by The Haworth Press, Inc.

Published 2019 by Routledge
2 Park Square, Milton Park, Abingdon, Oxon OX14 4RN
52 Vanderbilt Avenue, New York, NY 10017

Routledge is an imprint of the Taylor & Francis Group, an informa business

Infertility and Adoption: A Guide for Social Work Practice has also been published as *Journal of Social Work & Human Sexuality*, Volume 6, Number 1 1987.

Library of Congress Cataloging-in-Publication Data

Infertility and adoption.

"Journal of social work & human sexuality, Volume 6, Number 1."
Bibliography: p.
1. Adoption — United States. 2. Infertility — United States. 3. Family social work — United States. 4. Medical social work — United States. I. Valentine, Deborah.
HV875.55.I53   1988   362.7'34'0973   87-36635

ISBN 13: 978-0-86656-721-3 (hbk)

Dedication

To my family:

Gene, Jason, and Kesna Wells

and

To all persons involved in the rewards
and struggles of building a family

and

To a valued colleague
Donna P. Smith

ABOUT THE EDITOR

Deborah Valentine, MSSW, PhD, is Associate Professor at the University of South Carolina, College of Social Work in Columbia. She has been published on issues of child maltreatment, family violence, developmental processes of pregnancy and family relations. She has recently completed research projects investigating the emotional impact of infertility and factors associated with disrupted adoptive placements. Dr. Valentine is the Managing Editor of *Arete': Journal of the College of Social Work, University of South Carolina*.

Infertility and Adoption:
A Guide for Social Work Practice

CONTENTS

Contributors

Kenneth Burry, MD, Associate Professor of gynecology, reproductive endocrinology and infertility, Oregon Health Sciences University, School of Medicine in Portland, OR.

Patricia Conway, PhD, Associate Professor, College of Social Work, University of South Carolina, Columbia.

Sharon N. Covington, LCSW, Director of counseling and psychological services, Fertility Center, Rockville, MD.

Jeanne Fleming, PhD, Clinical Psychologist, private practice, Longview, WA.

Harold D. Grotevant, PhD, Associate Professor of child development and psychology, University of Texas, Austin, TX.

Ann Hartman, DSW, Dean and Elizabeth Marting Treuhaft Professor, Smith College of Social Work, Northhampton, MA.

Robert L. Howell, ACSW, Special Projects Administrator, South Carolina Department of Social Services, Columbia SC.

Page Townsend Johnson, MA, free-lance writer, Houston, TX.

Dorothy W. LePere, MSSW, Consultant and private practitioner, San Antonio, TX.

Ruth G. McRoy, PhD, Associate Professor, School of Social Work, University of Texas, Austin, TX.

Patricia Payne Mahlstedt, EdD, Clinical Instructor, Baylor College of Medicine, psychologist in private practice, Houston, TX.

Leroy H. Pelton, PhD, Professor, School of Social Work, Salem State College, Salem, MA.

Jerry Randolph, PhD, Associate Professor, College of Social Work, University of South Carolina.

Rita Rhodes, PhD, Instructor, Department of Neuropsychiatry and Behavioral Sciences, University of South Carolina, School of Medicine, SC.

Marietta E. Spencer, ACSW, Program Director, Post-Legal Adoption Services, Children's Home Society, St. Paul, MN.

Deborah Valentine, PhD, Associate Professor, College of Social Work, University of South Carolina.

Infertility and Adoption:
A Guide for
Social Work Practice

Foreword

In the pages of this journal, two areas of vital concern to individuals, families and social work practitioners are explored; infertility and adoption. Although these topics may appear to be only tangentially connected, in truth they are each related to and shaped by the powerful need and wish to build a family. The American value system has been intensely pro-family and pro-natalist. As so interestingly explored in Rita Rhodes' lead article, "Women, Motherhood, and Infertility," the social and historical content of pro-natalism has defined women without children as unfulfilled and undervalued, and families without children as deficient. The standard view of the family as a married couple with children born to them has defined all other family forms and ways of building a family as "less than," deviant, or even "improper" or "wrong." Although we have seen some shift in this position in recent years, values change slowly, and underneath the espoused acceptance of and support for alternate family forms lie critical attitudes that form the context within which people face infertility, attempt to develop fulfilling child-free lives, or build families through adoption.

Infertility and adoption are also connected in another way. Both have been considered to be areas of specialization, topics of concern only to those small groups of social workers practicing in adoption agencies or in medical settings specializing in fertility problems. The fact is that all social workers and other mental health professionals are in post-adoption practice, that professionals practicing in a wide variety of agencies will meet clients who have been faced with infertility. Every practitioner must have the knowledge and the skill to provide post-adoption services, to provide help around infertility. Further, every practitioner must become more aware of how widespread are adoption and infertility, so that they may recognize and deal with these important human concerns even when clients fail initially to identify them or recognize their salience.

The articles that follow are offered by specialists and bring to the social worker and other mental health practitioners the expertise and the knowledge to help these professionals become more sensitive to and competent in helping people around infertility and adoption.

We learn about the extent of infertility in the United States: one in every six couples of childbearing age is infertile, a 100% increase in 20 years. We learn how to evaluate the complex social and psychological transactions which develop around infertility and to become aware of the iatrogenic effects of insensitive handling by medical professionals. We learn the usefulness of knowledge and skills concerning crisis intervention, nurturing, and grief work with people experiencing reproductive loss. Finally, the crucial role of the infertile couple's intimate social network in coming to terms with infertility is explored.

Turning to adoption, Leroy Pelton describes this changing social institution. He spells out the radical social changes that have altered adoption from a program designed to place infants with young, infertile couples to one which aims to find a permanent family for all children in need of one, regardless of their age, or special physical or emotional needs. The tension between the growing number of infertile couples and the reduced availability of infants for adoption becomes clear as couples and unmarried adults search far and wide in their efforts to build a family. Extensive knowledge and skills are demanded of social workers who wish to help the new adoptive family in dealing with children with complex needs and problems. The outcomes of the lack of such knowledge and skill is painfully surfaced in Valentine, Conway, and Randolph's study of families who have suffered adoption disruptions.

Other changes in adoption have made practice with adoptees, birth parents and adoptive parents more demanding. For example, open adoptions help to heal distances and gaps in identity formation but complicate adoption practice. Finally, the growing awareness among all professionals that family building through adoption is indeed different than biological parenting makes it clear that at every age and particularly at every life transition, the adoptive family, the adopted child, or the adult adoptee may need skilled and sensitive help from a practitioner who understands adoption.

Although some adoption agencies are beginning to offer postadoption services beyond legalization, most help for the thousands of Americans who are in some way a part of the adoption triangle will be met by practitioners in a wide range of settings, by practitioners who must come to understand the meaning of adoption in the lives of the adoptive family, the adoptee, and the birth parent.

In the pages that follow, thoughtful and knowledgeable professionals respond to the need for special information to be disseminated to all practitioners who throughout the course of their practice will be called upon to serve clients suffering from reproductive loss and clients who have been intimately involved with adoption. There is a wealth of information here and it is for the practitioner to integrate this knowledge into more expert and sensitive helping.

Ann Hartman

Women, Motherhood, and Infertility: The Social and Historical Context

Rita Rhodes

SUMMARY. This article will consider varying societal responses to infertility over different periods of time. The role of religion, in particular, will be identified as a powerful influence on human behaviors surrounding fertility and infertility. The special consequences of infertility for women will also be examined. This historical perspective is useful in that deeply-rooted societal expectations continue to shape the fertility and infertility experiences of contemporary couples.

> Before all else, you are a wife and mother.
>
> *Henrik Ibsen*
> *A Doll's House*

> A race is worthless and contemptible if its men
> cease to be willing and able to work hard and,
> at need, to fight hard, and if its women cease
> to breed freely.
>
> *Theodore Roosevelt*

The social and historical significance of infertility is difficult to document and usually can only be studied indirectly, often by looking at its converse, fertility and motherhood. In an historical context, an examination of infertility also necessarily is limited by the nature of the material that is available. Because women more than men have been identified with their reproductive organs, the historical material that discusses fertility and causes of infertility is almost exclusively centered on the female experience. That female experience, moreover, is further restricted in that the women who were

5

discussed and studied were more likely to be white, middle class, and urban. A concentration on this limited population is not meant to suggest a unified experience of infertility by other classes, races and regions of the country. It can be argued, however, that writings about this group of women were held up as cultural norms against which other women might measure themselves.

COLONIAL PERIOD

In the New World during the 17th and 18th centuries, the majority of women married and their unions produced many children. A large family was an asset in a labor-intensive agricultural economy. Fertility was associated particularly with women. In the southern colonies, the boast was "Our land free, our men honest and our women fruitful" (Ryan, 1983). They were that, and colonial women of completed fertility had an average of eight children, making American fertility one of the world's highest (Grabill, Kiser & Whelpton, 1958:380).

The large number of pregnancies that women experienced in colonial America was fully consistent with their religious beliefs. The Plymouth Colony minister Cotton Mather, for example, associated pregnancy with the natural law created by God:

> It will be a very blamable Indecency and Indiscretion in you to be dissatisfied at your state of Pregnancy. . . . It will indeed look too unnatural in you to complain of a state whereunto the Laws of Nature, established by God had brought you.

Mather did not idealize pregnancy but rather insisted that "the griefs which you are now suffering in your Body are the Fruits of Sin" (Ryan, 1983). Mather's position was in keeping with the biblical association between pregnancy and sin:

> Adam was not deceived, but the woman was deceived
> and became a transgressor. Yet women will be saved
> through bearing children.

Timothy 2:14-15

Despite this acceptance that pain in childbirth was the logical consequence of female sinfulness, however, the colonial Puritans did not hold that infertile women were condemned to a lower level of spirituality. Indeed, Cotton Mather argued that "spinsters, widows, and those wives who were 'naturally barren' might find an easier path to 'Spiritual Fruitfulness . . . in all good works of Piety and Charity'" (Smith, 1970).

The worth of women beyond childbearing also is indicated in the Puritan attitude toward marriage. As valued as children were in colonial America, a marriage that produced no offspring was not sufficient cause for annulment. An exception to this, however, was impotence in the husband, and a divorce was granted in 1686 at Plymouth Colony to a woman who claimed that her husband was "always unable to perform the act of generation" (Demos, 1974). Although this description implies that the sexual act was intended for procreative purposes, childlessness was not grounds for divorce except perhaps when the source of infertility was obvious. When not obvious, a childless couple was not free to terminate their marriage in the hope of securing another spouse who might prove more fruitful.

In spite of the value assigned to the reproductive abilities of women, colonial America did not idealize motherhood. Indeed, childrearing was not the particular preserve of women but a task that was as likely to be assigned to older siblings, servants or neighbors. The idea that childhood was a special time with special requirements that were best provided by mothers was not part of the thinking of colonial Americans. The colonial image of woman was more likely to be based on her wide contributions to the survival of the family rather than on enhanced notions of motherhood. The labor of women was essential to the survival of the household and there existed few negative definitions of what was appropriate female work. The economic demands of colonial America blurred distinctions between the gender roles of men and women. As distressful a condition that childlessness might be for a colonial woman, she was not without value in a society that depended on women for the extensive work necessary for survival.

VICTORIAN PERIOD

By the middle of the 18th century, the subsistence economy of the colonial period was giving way to a commercial one. The social and economic roles of men and women were changing as the household declined as a unit of production and home and workplace became separate spheres. The compartmentalization of work and home was accompanied by a reevaluation of woman's role. New prescriptions for what was called "true womanhood" dictated that proper women limit their activities to the domestic sphere. For all women this new concept of femininity became an ideal even if its standards were unrealizable in their own lives.

This new ideal of femininity drew much stronger distinctions between proper male and female functions than had existed during the colonial period. In particular, the asexual colonial role of parenthood was replaced by an expanded concept of motherhood. The image of "woman as mother" became an increasingly accurate description as fewer economic activities were performed within the household. As late as the 1830s, there appeared the occasional "father's book," but by the middle of the century the primacy of motherhood was fully established.

During the rest of the Victorian period, the concept of motherhood became endowed with semisacred connotations while the significance of fatherhood continued its decline. *Harper's Bazaar*, for example, noted in 1900 that "the suburban husband and father is almost entirely a Sunday institution" (Filene, 1976). Motherhood had, in turn, moved to center stage and in 1914 a joint resolution passed by the entire United States Congress declared the second Sunday in May as Mother's Day. The resolution proclaimed the American mother as "the greatest source of the country's strength and inspiration" and described the results of her labor as "doing so much for the home, for moral uplift, and religion, hence so much for good government and humanity. . . . " (Filene, 1976).

This veneration of motherhood was part of a newly-established gender system which viewed men and women as having sharply different natures. For one New Haven professor it seemed "as if the Almighty, in creating the female sex, had taken the uterus and built up a woman around it" (Wood, 1974). Motherhood became the essence of femininity, and it was called "woman's one duty and function . . . that alone for which she was created" (Ryan, 1983). Women were considered at their most feminine when they were pregnant. Woman's reproductive ability was used to explain her special talents for parenting. The qualities that parenthood required — affection, caring, and patience — were linked exclusively to the female sex and considered part of the "maternal instinct." Many 19th century writings went so far as to view the maternal instinct as the female counterpart of the male sex instinct (Gordon, 1974).

Clearly associated with the notion of maternal instinct was the implication that women who did not become mothers remained unfulfilled. Even feminists such as Victoria Woodhull and Tennessee Claflin believed "that those who pass through life failing in this special feature (child bearing) of their mission cannot be said to have lived to the best purposes of woman's life" (Gordon, 1974). Both feminists and conservatives alike extolled motherhood as the essence of femininity. Infertile women not only were perceived as unfulfilled but also less feminine than other women.

The same reproductive organs that permitted a woman to enter the sacred state of motherhood also determined her physical and emotional health. According to one mid-19th century physician:

> Woman's reproductive organs are preeminent. They exercise a controlling influence upon her entire system, and entail upon her many painful and dangerous diseases. They are the source of her peculiarities, the centre of her sympathies, and the seat of her diseases. Everything that is peculiar to her, springs from her sexual organization. (Smith-Rosenberg, 1974)

As knowledge of woman's reproductive system expanded in the 19th century, the ovaries were identified as those agents that controlled the course of women's lives. A late 19th century physician described their significance:

> A woman's system is affected, we may almost say dominated, by the influence of these two little glands. . . . Either an excess or a deficiency of the proper influence of these organs over the other parts of the system may be productive of disease. (Smith-Rosenberg, 1974)

The extent to which a woman's reproductive organs dominated her life had no counterpart in the male.

It was held that irregularities in the functioning of the reproductive organs accounted for many female illnesses. A University of Pennsylvania professor in his text on the diseases of females argued that women were subject to twice the illnesses that affected men because of the uterus (Wood, 1974). It was believed, in turn, that infertile women were particularly vulnerable to insanity, cancer, and degenerative diseases (Harris, 1978). One physician accused his profession of adopting the attitude "if only she could have a child, it would cure her" (Wood, 1974). Infertile women encountered a medical profession that was likely to judge their condition as having far-reaching implications for their physical well-being.

Not only were women identified with their reproductive organs in the 19th century, but these organs did not appear to be functioning very well. The medical literature on the state of woman's health was gloomy enough for a Harvard medical professor to write: "It requires no prophet to foretell that the wives who are to be mothers in our republic must be drawn from transAtlantic homes" (Wood, 1974). The perceived increase in infertility among the native-born was blamed on the women themselves. Puberty was considered to be an especially dangerous period. How young women negotiated this phase was seen as indicative of the success or failure of their childbearing years.

For boys, the onset of puberty brought health, energy and strength, and the scope of activities believed appropriate for this age was enlarged. Feminine energy during adolescence, on the other hand, was believed to be at a premium as it was needed for the development of the reproductive organs. It was advised that pubescent girls restrict their activities. A psychologist, G. Stanley Hall, informed the National Education Association in 1903: "The first danger to woman is over-brainwork. It affects that part of her organism which is sacred to heredity." And a professor reported to the American Academy of Medicine in 1895 that the employed woman "commits a biologic crime against herself and the community. . . ." (Filene, 1976). Instead, physicians recommended a routine of domestic tasks that would conserve a young woman's energy and prepare her for her future in the domestic sphere. If an adolescent girl disregarded her female nature, "dysmenorrhea, miscarriage, even sterility" would follow (Smith-Rosenberg, 1974). A young girl (and her mother) had a responsibility to ensure a fertile future for herself.

During the Victorian period, men's and women's natures were perceived as very different. For women, biology was destiny and their reproductive function was presented as their most important function. Women's fertility was emphasized, and women were destined to devote themselves to motherhood, a task for which they were clearly designed. The belief that motherhood was a woman's fulfillment also had a material basis as economic functions left the household. Motherhood remained as the most creative part of a woman's life and an important part of her self-esteem. Married women who were infertile were left in the undesirable position of being perceived as less feminine and with few socially-sanctioned activities to occupy them. In addition, infertile women were judged to have brought their condition upon themselves. And finally, the medical literature predicted a dire future for her because of her malfunctioning reproductive organs.

The Victorians associated sexual passion exclusively with the male. The decade of the 1920s brought a change in this perception in that there was a more general recognition that women as well as men were sexual beings. The Darwinist Havelock Ellis, in his bestselling work *Man and Woman*, argued that women were as sexually passionate as men, although he continued to maintain that women possessed a unique female nature that suited them to the domestic role and motherhood. Another important advocate of female sexuality was Margaret Sanger, who promoted birth control to liberate female sexuality while also insisting on the power of the maternal impulse. Sanger suggested that woman's "self-realization will come through a gradual assertion of her power in her own sphere rather than in that of men" (Kennedy, 1973). One historian has noted that "it became possible in the 1920s to simultaneously take a radical stand on sex and a conservative one on women's social role" (O'Neill, 1969). This "New Victorianism" of the first half of the 20th century recognized female sexuality while it continued to promote norms that were not very different from the 19th century cult of true womanhood. Despite their "sexual liberation" infertile women could not free themselves from the social identification of women with motherhood.

The new Victorianism sought to raise the standards for motherhood and homemaking. There were efforts to restructure education in order to prepare women for the complicated role they would assume in the home. Both secondary schools and colleges developed courses in home economics. Women's colleges increasingly came under attack for offering their students courses comparable to men's and not preparing women for their future roles as wives and mothers (Harris, 1978). In response to such criticisms, Vassar College in 1924 created the School of Euthenics whose purpose was to reroute "education for women along the lines of their chief interests and responsibilities, motherhood, and the home." A supporter of this school defined its purpose as "to raise motherhood to a profession worthy of (woman's) finest talents and greatest intellectual gifts" (Chafe, 1974). Such efforts by educators reinforced an image of woman primarily as wife and mother and left women who would not or could not take up that role, less prepared for an alternative one.

Women's magazines also focused on skills for homemaking and motherhood and presented the role of mother and housewife as the only suitable one for women. *McCall's*, for example, observed that it was only as a wife and mother that a woman could "arrive at her true eminence." Women were encouraged to think of their domestic duties as a rewarding profession and *The Ladies Home Journal* declared that "the creation and fulfillment of a successful home is a bit of craftsmanship that compares favorably with building a beautiful cathedral" (Chafe, 1974). Career women who violated these norms were singled out by the women's magazines as unfeminine.

THE DEPRESSION

The Depression of the 1930s also reinforced notions of women's proper role within the home. A National Education Association study in 1930-1931 which surveyed 1500 school systems reported that 77% refused to hire wives and 63% dismissed teachers if they married. Federal legislation from 1932-1937 prohibited more than one member of a family from working in the civil service. This legislation effectively restricted the employment of women in government. Public disapproval of women employed outside the home was reflected in a 1936 Gallup Poll in which 82% of respondents answered negatively to the question of whether married women should work if their husbands were employed. Gallup believed that he had "discovered an issue on which voters are about as solidly united as on any subject imaginable — including sin and hay fever." The future Secretary of Labor under Franklin Roosevelt, Frances Perkins, argued that any woman who could support herself without a job "should devote herself to motherhood and the home" (Chafe, 1974). Infertile women without this option were not free to enter the male sphere of work.

WORLD WAR II

From 1920 to 1940, the notion that women's place was in the home as wife and mother was strengthened. Pearl Buck declared in 1940 that "men and children have proceeded with the times, but women have not, and today the home is too peculiarly hers" (Chafe, 1974). In 1940, the percentage of women employed outside the home was what it had been in 1910. World War II changed all that. To fill the needs of the wartime economy and maintain a huge army, society turned to women. Whereas women previously had been criticized for leaving the domestic sphere, they now were praised for responding to their country's needs. By the end of the war, the female labor force had increased by 6.5 million and for the first time more wives were employed than single women. In 1943, Margaret Hickey, head of the Women's Advisory Committee to the War Manpower Commission, noted that "employers, like other individuals, are finding it necessary to weigh old values, old institutions, in terms of a world at war" (Chafe, 1974). The question remained: What would be the role of women in a world at peace?

At the conclusion of the war, a combination of fears about recession, the policy of giving jobs to veterans, and traditional notions about women's proper sphere led to massive layoffs of female workers. In the year following, 2.25 million women left their employment and another million were laid off. This loss of jobs, however, proved temporary, and by 1947 female employment was nearing wartime levels. Responding to the persistence of female employment in the postwar years, the director of the Women's Bureau, Frieda Miller, speculated as early as 1947 that the nation was "approaching a period when for women to work is an act of conformism." Indeed, the rate of female employment continued to increase in the postwar decades and by 1960 twice as many women were at work as in 1940 (Chafe, 1974). The domestic sphere remained a central focus of women's lives but it was no longer the only focus and infertile women, like their sisters, had employment options outside the home that had not existed before.

POST WORLD WAR II

Despite the radical change in the employment of women, the persistence of views about women's proper role continued into the postwar period. These views gained support from a new source after World War II — Freudian psychology. In the postwar decades, Freud's work was promoted and became an important influence on popular culture. Freudianism supported the notion of a separate female sphere in the scientific terminology of the 20th century. Freud, like the good Victorian that he was, made biological differences the center piece of his theory in explaining male and female psychic development. A girl deprived of a penis substituted for it a desire to bear her father's child; in the healthy adult woman this desire was transferred to another male. If adult women did not seek to become mothers, "they were suffering from unresolved penis envy and a masculinity complex" (Harris, 1978).

An important disciple of Freud who more fully developed a Freudian position on women was Helene Deutsch, whose study *The Psychology of Women* was published in 1944. This work became a bible for psychoanalytic practitioners with a female clientele and gave new support to the cult of motherhood. Deutsch argued that even female sexuality was part of the desire for motherhood: "In the normal healthy woman coitus psychologically represents the first act of motherhood." She encouraged fertility as natural and as a protection against psychic damage in women: "having many children is the best protection against this tragic loss" (Ryan, 1983). An infertile woman, therefore, in this analysis presumably would suffer psychological damage.

Deutsch's work, in turn, was popularized in a best-selling work by Ferdinand Lundberg and Marynia Farnham entitled *Modern Women: The Lost Sex*. A pitfall of modern society, they suggested, was the confusion of male and female roles. Modern women had lost sight of the scientific truth that women are:

> endowed with a complicated reproductive system with which the male genitourinary system compares in complexity not at all, a more elaborate nervous system and an infinitely complex psychology revolving about the reproductive function. Women, therefore, cannot be regarded as any more similar to men than a spiral is to a straight line. (Smith, 1970)

Lundberg and Farnham argued that motherhood was a cornerstone for healthy psychic development and that one of the ills of the 20th century was the failure on the part of women to accept motherhood as the ultimate goal of their lives (Harris, 1978). Female happiness could be ensured by the acceptance of women's biologically-determined role as mother. In this world view, "anatomy is destiny" and one was either a well-adjusted homemaker/mother or a feminist neurotic.

During the decade of the 1950s it appeared that the gender system supported by the Freudians was working quite well. The rapid development of suburbs expressed in concrete the separate spheres for men and women. Within their sphere, women were becoming devoted to motherhood as they had not done before and a larger proportion of women became mothers than at any other time in American history. These women not only married and began childbearing at an earlier age than their mothers and grandmothers, they also had more children than these two generations. Between 1940 and 1960 the birthrate for third children doubled and that for fourth children tripled (Chafe, 1974). The sheer number of births ensured a cultural preoccupation with motherhood and fertility.

Women's magazines reflected this postwar preoccupation with maternity and essentially proclaimed that "motherhood is a way of life." Advertisers in magazines and television targeted women as mothers and homemakers who would make increasing purchases for their expanding families. *Fortune* magazine attributed the healthy business climate to the fact that more "nubile females are marrying than ever before." And when the economy weakened during the recession of 1957, *Life* magazine proclaimed: "Kids — Built-in Recession Cure — How four million a year make millions in business" (Ryan, 1983). When women saw themselves portrayed in the media it was more often than not in the garb of motherhood. Infertile women were surrounded by the trappings of a pronatalist society.

Not surprisingly, women also defined themselves as mothers and homemakers. In a 1967 survey of 15,000 college women, 57% agreed or agreed strongly with the statement, "Having children is the most important function of marriage." And that percentage arguably would have been increased if the statement had been rephrased "Having children is among the most important functions of marriage" (Gordon, 1978). In a 1962 Gallup poll, 90% of women called childbirth the "most satisfying moment" of their lives (Chafe, 1974). Women also appeared more anxious to repeat those moments. In 1945, 31% of white women thought the ideal number of children was four; a decade later that had increased to 41% (Filene, 1976). College women did not appear to diverge from these views and a 1961 Smith College student newspaper editorialized: "Perhaps we are old-fashioned but we feel that for the majority of women, their place is 'in the home'" (Filene, 1976). Infertile women would have good cause to feel estranged from the female experience of their generation.

In 1963 Betty Friedan published an attack on this view of women in a book that sold over a million copies, *The Feminine Mystique*. It was Friedan's thesis that after 1949 women had been restricted to only one definition for themselves, as the housewife-mother. The "feminine mystique" emphasized the differences between men and women and urged women to accept "their own nature which can find fulfillment only in sexual passivity, male domination, and nurturing maternal love" (Friedan, 1970). Friedan argued that the mystique found an easy acceptance in the climate of postwar America where those who had experienced depression and war now sought "the comforting reality of home and children" (Friedan, 1970). She blamed the pervasiveness of the mystique on Freudian psychoanalytic theory, women's magazines, advertisers, function-

alist social scientists, and educators. For Friedan, the internaliza-
tion of the mystique stunted the growth of women who made no
plans outside of marriage and maternity.

The problem that Friedan presented as originating in the postwar
climate, however, did not differ dramatically from the "cult of true
womanhood" that had permeated the 19th century. The fact that the
problem was reexamined and received such a positive reception was
related to the social climate of the 1960s, when the grievances of
oppressed minorities were beginning to be recognized. The analo-
gies that women drew between their position and that of minorities,
together with the economic fact that women were already challeng-
ing a basic premise of the mystique by their increasing employment
outside the home, accounted, in part, for the responsive chord
struck by the *Feminine Mystique*. The feminists who followed
Friedan challenged the notion of separate spheres and demanded a
role for women beyond their reproductive functions.

The demographic experience of the 1970s and 1980s indicates
that the reality of women's lives was diverging rapidly from the
ideology of separate spheres for men and women. In 1980 over 50%
of women aged 20 to 24 were single; and unmarried women in their
late 20s accounted for nearly 30% of their age group, a percentage
increase that was nearly double that of 1970. In addition, "the percentage of 30-year-old women who were childless rose from a postwar high of 14% in 1969 to almost 26% ten years later" (Ryan,
1983). The notion that women should remain in the domestic sphere
and devote themselves exclusively to motherhood was being challenged by increasing numbers of women. Clearly, the route to feminine fulfillment no longer lay solely in fertility and motherhood.

While the 1960s and 1970s produced a widespread criticism of
the gender system, the late 1970s and 1980s saw the emergence of
those dedicated to preserving the "traditional" family. The anxi-
eties about family life were articulated by a variety of commentators. The well-known author Michael Novak, for example, stated
his concerns in an article in *Harper's* in 1976:

> Choosing to have a family used to be uninteresting. It is today,
> an act of intelligence and courage. To love family life, to see
> in family life the most potent moral, intellectual, and political

cell in the body politic is to be marked today as a heretic. (Gordon, 1978)

The defense of the family and older gender roles has been taken up as a particular cause of the New Right. The influence of the New Right has increased with the election of Ronald Reagan, a man with conservative views on gender and the family. Senator Paul Laxalt, for example, introduced in Congress "The Family Protection Act" in which federal funds would be denied for schoolbooks or programs which "belittle the traditional role of women in society" (Ryan, 1983). This "traditional" position also was defended by authors such as Marabel Morgan, who in her best-selling work *Total Womanhood* sought to reassure women on the continuing validity of the domestic role.

The changing attitudes of the 1960s and 1970s also were identified by some professionals as a possible source of psychogenic infertility in women. A physician reasoned:

> If psychogenic infertility exists, (it) must be seen within the general context of the present social turmoil, with its accompanying upheaval of sexual values, unrestrained expression of feeling by the women's liberation movement, decrease in fertility rates, and general questioning of values with regard to families. (Denber, 1978)

Women with aspirations that had been encouraged by the social climate of the 1960s and 1970s encountered professionals who held that infertility was frequently psychogenic and due to stress between professional and maternal commitments. A professional in an infertility clinic argued that position:

> Sterility can thus be a defence of the disturbed personality against the experience of pregnancy and motherhood. The equality of the sexes, which our present-day society fosters, tends to make woman less submissive and her ego appears to be stronger; she has aspirations which may indeed be in conflict with the function of reproduction. (Sandler, 1968)

Infertile women were indicted for their participation in the advances made by their sex in the postwar decades.

Established feminists also appear moved by the fears of family breakdown and are reconsidering earlier positions on gender roles. Alice Rossi, a sociologist whose initial writings had challenged restrictive gender roles, wrote in 1977 on the "instinctual basis for mother-child bonding" (Ryan, 1983). Rossi argued that the family was best protected by strengthening the biological ties between women and children. Betty Friedan also responded to the perceived family crisis in a subsequent work entitled *The Second Stage*. Friedan's focus had moved from the isolated mother/housewife to the conflicted career woman who was struggling with the choice to have children. Friedan warned against the feminist mystique:

> To deny the part of one's being as woman that has, through the ages, been expressed in motherhood — nurturing, loving softness, and tiger strength — is to deny part of one's personhood as a woman. I am not saying that everyone has to be a mother to 'fulfill' herself as a woman. (Friedan, 1981)

By implication, however, Friedan did suggest that the majority of women do need motherhood in order to achieve fulfillment. The power of the maternal image of women is such that it continues to exert a strong influence on both feminists and conservatives alike.

CONCLUSION

In this overview of women, infertility, and motherhood in America, it has been suggested that notions of femininity have fluctuated and that three distinct gender patterns can be identified. During the colonial period women had a central role in the economy and the demands of the New World were such that notions about a distinct female nature and temperament were not advanced. The early 19th century marked a transition from this gender system to one based on a sexual division of labor. During this period, gender roles were particularly polarized and women were perceived primarily as mothers. Finally, since the 1960s there appears to have been a restructuring of the gender system that contains the potential for the full social integration of women into the work force. It can be suggested that those historical periods that define women as biologically distinct and suited primarily to motherhood, the infertile woman had a more difficult time securing a positive image for herself. The extent to which societal values acknowledge a role for women beyond reproduction is an index of the regard that infertile women can expect from the larger society.

REFERENCES

Chafe, W.H. (1974). *The American woman: Her changing social, economic, and political roles*, 1920-1970. New York: Oxford University Press.

Demos. J. (1974). *A little commonwealth: Family life in plymouth colony*. New York: Oxford University Press.

Denber, H.C.B. (1978). Psychiatric aspects of infertility. *Journal of Reproductive Medicine, 20* (1), 23-29.

Filene, P.G. (1976). *Him/her/self: Sex roles in modern America*. New York: New American Library, Mentor Books.

Friedan, B. (1970). *The feminine mystique*. New York: Dell Publishing.

Friedan, B. (1981). *The second stage*. New York: Summit Books.

Gordon, L. (1974). Voluntary motherhood: he beginnings of feminist birth control ideas in the United States. In M. Hartman & L. W. Banner (Eds.), *Clio's consciousness raised*. New York: Harper Torchbooks.

Gordon, M. (1978). *The American family: Past, present and future*. New York: Random House.

Grabill, W.; Kiser, C. & Whelpton, C. (1958). *The fertility of American Women*. New York: John Wiley and Sons.

Harris, B.J. (1978). *Beyond her sphere: Women and the professions in American history*. Westport, CT: Greenwood Press.

Kennedy, D.M. (1973). *Birth control in America*. New Haven: Yale University Press.

O'Neill, W.L. (1969). *Everyone was brave: The rise and fall of feminism in the United States*. Chicago: Quadrangle Books.

Ryan, M. (1983). *Womanhood in America*. New York: Franklin Watts.

Sandler, B. (1968). Emotional stress and infertility. *Journal of Psychosomatic Research, 12*, 51-59.

Smith, P. (1970). *Daughters of the promised land*. Boston: Little, Brown & Company.

Smith-Rosenberg, C. (1974). Puberty to menopause: The cycle of femininity in nineteenth-century America. In M. Hartman & L. Banner (Eds.), *Clio's consciousness raised*. New York: Harper Torchbooks.

Wood, A.D. (1974). The fashionable diseases: Women's complaints and their treatment in nineteenth-century America. In M. Hartman & L. Banner (Eds.), *Clio's consciousness raised*. New York: Harper Torchbooks.

Psychosocial Evaluation
of the Infertile Couple:
Implications for Social Work Practice

Sharon N. Covington

SUMMARY. The fields of medicine and social work have grown progressively closer over the years as the interrelatedness of the physical and psychosocial aspects of illness have become known. Infertility treatment requires the same integrated approach. This paper will focus on a model for the psychosocial evaluation of infertility patients as developed by the author. Case examples from the author's clinical experiences will be presented to illustrate the model. The implications for social work within the infertility medical practice will be discussed.

Social work has long been involved with medical patient care, primarily in hospitals. Social workers have helped patients and their families adjust to medical conditions by providing support, understanding, and resources. Medical social work has grown with the awareness of the psychosocial component of physical illness. Within medicine, there is an increasing recognition of psychological factors in the etiology, course, and treatment of disease. Mental health practitioners, including psychiatric social workers, have used their skills to help modify and change behaviors of medical patients while working in a primary care (ambulatory office or group) practice (Cooper et al, 1975; Mechnic, 1980).

As patients have become more psychologically sophisticated, they have become more motivated to seek care for the associated distress of their medical problems. We hear the term holistic medicine used to indicate the practice integration of all patient needs — physical, psychological, social, and spiritual. Additionally, social workers no longer identify themselves by practice setting (e.g., medical or psychiatric), but by a broader term indicating training area (e.g., clinical). The emerging field of medical psychotherapy, finds the psychotherapist working in the health care field be it the hospital, specialty clinic, or physician's office (Staff, 1986). Today, clinical social workers are found in such varied primary medical care settings as kidney dialysis centers, neurology clinics, oncology practices, and reproductive medical groups.

CLINICAL SOCIAL WORK
AND REPRODUCTIVE MEDICINE

Infertility, the inability to conceive or to carry a pregnancy to term, is an increasing medical problem. It is experienced by one of every six couples of childbearing age and affects almost ten million men and women — twice as many as 20 years ago. This is more people than inhabit the state of Michigan. Female factors account for approximately 40% of infertility, male factors another 40% and combined male/female factors, or unknown causes, for 20%. Infertility is a growing problem related to changing life styles, delayed childbearing, and complications from contraception and disease. Medical evaluation involves such procedures as physical examination of the body, particularly the genitals and reproductive organs; hormonal testing, through blood samples or radiological procedures; and investigation of sexual habits and behaviors, such as frequency of coitus, technique and orgasmic performance. Medical treatment may involve surgical repair of the genitals and reproductive organs; drug therapy which can be time-consuming, expensive, and uncomfortable; and/or physical intervention which encourages conception, such as artificial insemination or invitro fertilization.

The interrelationship between the medical and psychological components of fertility problems have been established in the literature (Christie, 1980; Keye, 1984; Mahlstedt, 1980; Menning, 1980; Seibel & Taymor, 1982). The very nature of the testing and treatment process is physically and psychologically intrusive. Patients can experience anxiety, pain, and emotional trauma as their bodies are touched, poked, and prodded. A couple's sex life, a very sensitive subject, is thoroughly probed, examined, and recorded. Patients often feel inadequate and defective, whether or not a diagnosis is made. This can be reinforced by medical terminology that describes reproductive functioning as hostile (cervical mucous), incompetent (cervix), defective (luteal phase), or poor (semen). Patients may feel distressed and frustrated by the medical process and by the insensitivity of medical caregivers. Extreme stress can effect hormone balances and endocrine functioning. Thus, psychological stress can become both the cause and effect of infertility (Sorrel & DeCherney, 1985).

The need for psychological support for infertile couples has been addressed by a number of authors (Batterman, 1985; Berger, 1977; Bresnick, 1981; Kraft et al., 1980; Mazor, 1979; Menning, 1977; Shapiro, 1982). At the very least, counseling, in conjunction with medical treatment, serves to enhance the quality of life of infertility patients (Bresnick & Taymor, 1979). At the very most, psychotherapeutic intervention may increase the chance for pregnancy (Sorrel & DeCherney, 1985). However, there is little hard scientific data in the literature to indicate the effectiveness of psychotherapeutic intervention with infertile patients. Most studies are lacking the necessary rigorous research design (Ellsworth & Shain, 1985; Fein, 1985). More scientific research needs to be done in this area.

Historically, social work with infertile couples probably began with adoption. The child was seen as the client, and counseling focused on the couple's ability to parent. Little recognition was given to the infertile couple's needs for psychological support (Menning, 1975). Today, infertility has become a human condition that often requires social work intervention. Infertility is a medical problem that permeates all aspects of a couple's life—body, mind, personality, and relationships. It is difficult, and indeed, inappropriate to separate the medical from the emotional aspects of the problem.

Clinical social workers need to have the unique knowledge and skills necessary to assess the needs of infertile couples. This encompasses two areas—the medical and the psychological. Medical knowledge includes a familiarity with the terminology; the knowledge of standard medical treatment and advances in the area of infertility treatment; and an understanding of what occurs physically and emotionally during specific testing and procedures. Psychological knowledge includes the application of crisis, bereavement, and ego development theory to the unique aspects of infertility. Many social workers in this field, like the author, began to obtain this knowledge from their personal experience with fertility problems.

THE LIFE CRISIS OF IMPAIRED FERTILITY

Reproduction is viewed as one of the most primal and basic of all human needs. In today's technocratic world, few couples ever anticipate any difficulty in having a baby. If they are unable to conceive or carry a baby, a crisis situation occurs. Infertility is an unanticipated crisis in the developmental life cycle of the family.

Theorists identify a crisis as any event which is seen by an individual as a threat, loss, or challenge of a life goal. The event is felt as a stress which may seem insolvable and beyond usual coping mechanisms. A period of psychological disequilibrium with associated high anxiety ensues. This may awaken key unresolved issues from the near and distant past. The crisis is a time-limited situation which creates a turning point for psychological regression or growth (Linderman, 1965; Rapoport, 1962).

Menning (1980) was the first author to write specifically about the infertility life crisis. She noted that infertility created a block to the developmental task of procreation and generativity. A person's motivation for pregnancy and parenthood, whether conscious or unconscious, is threatened and needs to be explored for resolution to occur. These motivations may relate to societal pressures and role fulfillment; a psychological rite of passage to adulthood; a desire for genetic continuity; proof of femininity or masculinity; and the need to replay or rework issues from the past, such as childhood or a failed pregnancy.

The infertility crisis reflects a multifaceted loss. Mahlstedt (1980) identified that infertility involves a loss in eight different areas. These include losses of relationships (both real and fantasy), health, status, self-esteem, confidence, security, and hope. She notes that in other life experiences: "Any *one* of these losses could precipitate a depressive reaction in an adult. The experience of infertility involves them *all*."

   The feelings of loss are experienced as a grief reaction, similar to the mourning process described by Batterman (1985), Mazor (1979), and Shapiro (1982) in their work with infertile couples. As a couple becomes aware of the infertility, they may feel surprised and *shocked*. One partner may *deny* the existence of the problem as a defense to the anticipation of overwhelming feelings. The emotional realization of the infertility problem generates intense feelings. Couples feel *angry* about the loss of control over their bodies and life choices. The anger is a reflection of feeling helpless and powerless toward infertility. It may be directed outward at physicians, family, friends, and God. Or the anger may be directed inward at self and become *depression*. The more difficulty a couple has in dealing with the anger and depression, the more socially isolated they become. As patients look inward and try to understand why this is happening to them, they often feel *guilty*. This is particularly true for the partner who is identified as having the problem. They may blame themselves for past decisions and behaviors, such as prior sexual relationships, contraception methods, or an abortion. The final phase of grieving, *resolution*, occurs when the loss of the wished for child is psychologically accepted and no longer is the focus of all emotional energy. It is only at this point that infertile couples can appropriately make decisions on other alternatives like adoption, artificial insemination by donor, or remaining child-free.

   Grief is the emotional response to a loss, and mourning is the process used to come to terms with the loss. It is here a distinction should be made between those couples who are unable to conceive and those couples who have been unable to successfully carry a pregnancy (miscarriage and stillbirth). Although the feelings of grief are similar, the mourning process may differ. A failed pregnancy is an *acute* situation due to the sudden and unexpected nature of the loss. However, the inability to conceive is often a more *chronic* situation. The loss emerges slowly over time as the couple identifies the problem, seeks treatment, and looks for solutions. For some couples, the process may take years with no diagnosis or effective treatment.

   Some couples experience both difficulty in conceiving and carrying a pregnancy, which precipates what this author terms "double-barreled grief." These couples feel betrayed and doubly wounded, as their elation from the wished for pregnancy has turned to profound grief. They must grieve for their dead baby, while wondering if they will ever become pregnant again. It is a formidable task. One woman who had an ectopic pregnancy after ten years of infertility treatment grieved intensely for many months over the loss of her baby. She poignantly reflected that she did not want to stop grieving as it was her only tie to this baby. Resolving her grief would mean letting go of the biological child she may never again have.

The mourning process presents unique difficulties for infertile couples. First, the loss is not evident to other people. It is the loss of hopes, dreams, and fantasies of a child that isn't visible to other people. Second, it is a loss that can't be easily communicated. One man commented, "Talking about infertility is like Victorian sex. Nice people don't do it!" The loss is felt as a personal failure, a narcissistic injury, that is not easy to share with other people. Also, since infertility relates to sex, many people feel that it is inappropriate and uncomfortable to discuss it. Lastly, there are no socially acceptable avenues for mourning this loss. There are no wakes, funerals, or religious services for infertility. Couples find themselves grieving a loss which is not acknowledged or validated by society. There is a sense that this experience has changed their lives forever, and yet it seems inconsequential to the rest of the world. The result is that infertile couples often find themselves experiencing intense emotions in virtual isolation.

The infertility experience is psychically traumatic, creating a threat to a patient's *sense of self*. In ego development theory, the psychic structure of "self" forms very early in life. The ego reflects feelings people have about their bodies *(body-image)* and how they see themselves in relation to others *(self-image)*. Infertility patients suffer narcissistic injury from blows to both self-image and body-image. The medical process focuses on failure, for if they had "succeeded" they wouldn't be there. Patients feel that their bodies, the very essence of who they are, are defective and have failed them. They may feel ashamed of their bodies, lose interest in sex, or have difficulty performing on schedule. Infertility is equated with a sense of sexual failure since they cannot "make a baby."

The assault on a patient's self-esteem, self-confidence, and sexuality can be devastating.

THE PSYCHOSOCIAL EVALUATION OF INFERTILE COUPLES

The framework for the psychosocial evaluation of the infertile couple was developed by this author while in a private reproductive medical practice. The practice is made up of gynecologists, urologists, endocrinologists, psychotherapists, nurses, laboratory technicians and administrative staff. The philosophy of the practice is that: (1) the evaluation and treatment of infertility demands a unified approach and (2) the medical and emotional aspects of infertility cannot be separated. The identified patient is a triad—husband, wife, and couple—who is seen as part of this team approach. The first appointment for the couple consists of a detailed review of medical history and physical examination with the gynecologist and urologist, followed by a counseling session with the social worker. A physician participates in the first few minutes of the session by introducing the couple and giving a brief overview of the medical history, results of the physical examination, and projected course of treatment. This beginning reinforces the idea of a team, which encourages open communication.

The social worker becomes a supportive communication link between physician, patient, and staff. The session provides the social worker with the opportunity to give the couple concrete information on the medical and emotional aspects of infertility and ways to cope with the stress. In addition, the session provides the social worker with the opportunity to learn from the couple additional information which may be useful to the medical staff. Infertile couples can begin to acknowledge feelings about their limitations, while focusing on their strengths. If significant psychosocial problems are evident during the evaluation or if they occur during medical treatment, counseling and psychotherapy are provided by the social worker as an integrated part of the practice. The message to the couple is that they will be physically and emotionally supported throughout the process, thereby minimizing the inherent stresses of medical evaluation and treatment.

Method

The purpose of the psychosocial evaluation is to assess the couple's functioning in relation to their fertility problem. Thus, this framework can be used in any practice setting (e.g., adoption agency or mental health clinic) where there is a need to evaluate the effect of infertility on psychosocial functioning. The evaluation involves three activities for the social worker: assessment, interpretation, and intervention. *Assessment activities* require the social worker to evaluate psychosocial functioning of the couple, at present and prior to infertility treatment. *Interpretive activities* involve communicating to the medical staff the psychosocial issues unique to this patient and helping the patient understand the medical terminology, evaluation and treatment process. *Interventive activities* involve the use of psychotherapeutic techniques to change behavior.

Assessment Activities

The interview provides the opportunity for the social worker to evaluate the psychosocial functioning of the couple. It is important to look for a distinction between how the couple functioned before the recognition of infertility versus the present. The three areas considered are:

Biological factors. This area includes medical, sexual, and health history. Some of the questions that need to be answered are: Have there been other medical treatments in the past, related or unrelated to infertility? How did they feel about it? Are sexual problems new or did they exist before infertility? What has their physical health been like in the past versus today? What is their use of alcohol and recreational drugs?

Psychological factors. This includes psychiatric history and ego development, which can provide answers to these questions: Is there any familial history of psychiatric problems? Have they ever been involved in counseling or psychotherapy? What were the circumstances? How has this couple coped in the past with problems? What ego losses have they experienced in the past? What is their self-image and body-image now versus before infertility? What is their mood, memory, thought process, and perception like?

Social factors. This includes history of primary family, marriage, friendship, employment, education, religion, and cultural background. Some areas that need to be explored are: What has their relationship been like with their primary family? Have there been prior marriages, and how does this affect them (stepfamily issues)? What is their career/job satisfaction? How has the job been affected by infertility? What kind of a support system do they have? Are they able to use it? How does their religious, cultural, or ethnic background affect infertility feelings? What is the significance of a child in their lives?

Interpretive Activities

The psychosocial interview can serve as the bridge between the medical and psychological issues of infertility. The patient may need help in understanding medical terminology and the evaluation/treatment process. Whether or not patients are medically unsophisticated or have limited educational backgrounds, they may feel too uncomfortable to ask the doctor questions. Never assuming the couple's knowledge, the social worker explores their understanding of pertinent medical information, providing explanations or referring back to the physician. For example, a professional couple in which the wife was a nurse, was unclear about the timing and positioning of coitus. They were too embarrassed to ask the physician, since they felt their "ignorance" would reflect negatively to the doctor.

Frequently, the interview uncovers new medical and psychological information from the couple which may be useful to the medical staff. For example, anxiety from prior painful medical experiences can be debilitating or block treatment. During one interview, a woman stated that she had abruptly stopped evaluation with another physician after a painful endometrial biopsy. She was ashamed of this, yet fearful of another biopsy. The team was alerted and extra support given to help her with any invasive testing.

Interventive Activities

Although the psychosocial evaluation usually is a single interview, the opportunity exists for intervention to change behavior. Psychotherapeutic techniques might include identification, clarification and interpretation of feelings, coping strategies, and anxiety – or stress-reducing skills. Examples of some coping strategies are appropriate avoidance of painful situations (e.g., baby showers), limit setting (e.g., restricting talk about infertility to 20 minutes a day), goal setting (e.g., a time frame for treatment), exploring alternatives while continuing treatment (e.g., adoption workshops), and generating emotional support (e.g., joining a support group). Stress-reducing skills can focus on relaxation techniques and imaging exercises. Short-term counseling or psychotherapy can be offered when the couple manifests significant stress or psychopathology which cannot be dealt with during the evaluation.

Intervention can be both *restorative* and *preventative*, depending on how long the couple has identified themselves as infertile. The newly identified couple may have just begun to question if they have a fertility problem when they seek medical advice. They are usually under less stress, may resent being called infertile, and can use intervention to help prevent problems. The long-term identified couple may have been undergoing evaluation and treatment for a long time, and they may have seen many different doctors. They are usually under significant stress, have acquiesced to being called infertile, and can use intervention to help restore their functioning.

Objectives

The framework for the psychosocial infertility evaluation includes four objectives.

To Assess the Couple's Relationship and Discuss Current Concerns About the Infertility Problem

The first step in any evaluation is to help the couple to talk about their relationship and how this crisis is affecting it. Discussing how the couple feels about the medical evaluation/treatment plan, leads the social worker to a better understanding of how infertility has affected their feelings about themselves, their marriage, and other relationships. The social worker should look for the degree of mutuality, supportiveness, and creativity within the marriage as well as within the individual. This should be evaluated within the context of how the couple was coping before infertility and how the couple is coping now. The couple needs reassurance that many of their feelings are normal and appropriate for this stressful situation. However, even when a couple is expressing a normal response to infertility, further intervention may be useful to avoid potential problems.

Abnormal reactions requiring further intervention are a matter of degree and duration of symptoms. They include: feelings of sadness and depression that are making it difficult to find any pleasure in life; anxiety that is overpowering daily functioning and concentration; significant change in sleeping or eating habits; lack of supportiveness, conflicts, or blaming behavior between the couple; excessive dependency needs or excessive overachieving; sexual difficulties, especially performance; serious employment problems, social isolation, or loss of friendships.

To Evaluate Possible Psychological Hindrances to the Medical Treatment Process

Infertility is not a psychiatric illness. The incidence of psychosomatic infertility is extremely low, while the resulting stress is extremely high. However, psychological resistances may occur which make it difficult to provide effective medical treatment. These resistances are often manifested by ambivalence or undermining behavior to suggested treatment. They may include such instances as frequently forgetting to take a basal body temperature or medication; procrastination around a semen analysis; "doctor hopping" without completing testing; and not following through on suggested medical procedures. For example, a man who was discovered to have a low sperm count was told by the physician to stop smoking marijuana, a known factor in male infertility. During the psychosocial evaluation, they were asked how they felt about what the doctor had said. The man shared that he didn't believe the doctor and wasn't going to follow the instructions. Without this knowledge and appropriate intervention by the team, his behavior and denial of responsibility could undermine treatment.

To Anticipate Problems that Can Occur During the Medical Evaluation and Discuss Ways of Coping with the Stress

An underlying assumption in the psychosocial infertility evaluation is that the more information and knowledge a couple has about the medical and emotional components of fertility treatment, the better able the couple is to cope with problems and stress as they occur. This helps the couple feel more in control about what is happening to their bodies and their lives. Anticipation can aid in prevention. The social worker can educate the couple about some of the problems couples encounter during medical evaluation and coping mechanisms can be suggested. This can help them feel more normal about their responses and avert more severe problems.

For example, the couple may begin to develop sexual problems due to the demand nature of ovulatory coitus. They may need to allow themselves a "vacation" from infertility and scheduled sex or be given other suggestions on ways to make sexual relations more pleasurable. Other problems which can be anticipated include anxiety over medical procedures, such as laparoscopy; diminished self-esteem and self-image; isolation from or discomfort with family, friends, and certain social occasions, such as parties with pregnant women and children; rekindled old hurts from the past; the emotional rollercoaster of the menstrual/ovulatory cycle, that is anticipation, hope, and despair; and general stress responses.

To Provide Information and Education on Infertility

The fourth objective of the psychosocial infertility evaluation is to provide information on support resources and reading materials. Every couple should be made aware of RESOLVE, a self-help organization for infertile people. Books on the medical and emotional aspects of infertility are also useful. Articles on specific concerns or procedures should be made available, such as AID (artificial insemination by donor), IVF (in vitro fertilization), GIFT (Gamete Intra-Fallopian Transfer), hormonal medications, surgical treatments, and coping issues. Finally, the couple should be made aware that the social worker is a resource for information on alternatives to biological parenthood, such as adoption and childfree living.

These four objectives should be covered in a way that focuses on the couple's strengths and mental health. The medical evaluation process tends to make the couple feel ineffective, defective, and out of control. The psychosocial evaluation provides an opportunity to help the couple put some control and health back in their lives.

The psychosocial infertility evaluation will provide a basis for recommending further psychological support. Reading materials and joining RESOLVE should be encouraged for all patients. No formal services may be needed for couples who seem to be coping adequately and have an integrated support system. Support groups or counseling may be helpful for psychologically healthy couples who have become socially isolated and are having difficulty coping. Psychotherapy may be appropriate for psychologically wounded couples where infertility is just an additional struggle in already difficult lives. For these couples, infertility can be their "calling card" for therapy. Recommendations for further help should focus on the positive aspect of the opportunity available for change due to the life crisis of infertility.

CASE STUDY

Mr. and Mrs. R. were seen at The Fertility Center for an initial counseling session following gynecologic and urologic evaluation. The R.'s had been attempting pregnancy for six months, when they consulted Mrs. R.'s gynecologist. Preliminary testing indicated mild endometriosis and a luteal phase defect, which was treated with progesterone suppositories. When they were still not pregnant one year later, the R.'s wanted a second opinion. Neither had any unusual medical problems prior to infertility. Mrs. R.'s initial physical examination was normal, and further hormonal testing was initiated. However, Mr. R. had a borderline semen analysis and a varicocele was discovered on examination. Further urologic follow-up was indicated to determine if surgical repair was warranted.

The R.'s had been married seven years but had known each other for 11 years. Mr. R., 34 and an engineer, was a quiet, slightly built man who appeared distracted through much of the interview. Mrs. R., a 32-year-old school teacher, was an attractive woman who initially seemed tense and controlled. However, she started to cry as she described their struggles in trying to have a baby. She quickly apologized for her tears, saying her husband was "much better" at handling his feelings than she was. Mrs. R.'s job, which had always been a source of satisfaction for her, was becoming a problem. She was tired of taking care of other peoples' children, felt stagnant, but had continued to teach as she saw it as a good occupation for a working mother.

Mrs. R. came from a large, Irish Catholic family, and was the only sibling who didn't have children. She felt supported in the past by her family and friends but now felt no one understood her feelings of inadequacy because they could have babies so easily. Mr. R. remained distant as his wife cried. He described himself as "not very close" to his family, who live in another state. When asked how the infertility was affecting him, he said that it didn't really matter to him if they had a baby but he wanted his wife to be happy. He said that he was skeptical of the practice of medicine, and felt they shouldn't "tamper with Mother Nature." Mrs. R. became angry with this comment. The R.'s felt that their sexual relationship was no longer enjoyable and at times wonder "why bother if we can't make a baby."

Impressions: the R.'s are experiencing many of the stresses couples feel as they undergo medical evaluation. Frustration with the medical process, loss of sexual pleasure, feelings of inadequacy, dissatisfaction with job, and a growing emotional isolation from family, friends, and each other. Although these feelings are normal for infertile couples, the situation could become critical without supportive intervention. Prior to infertility, the R.'s were functioning adequately. However, Mr. R.'s emotional withdrawal and Mrs. R.'s increasing anxiety and depression were beginning to cause marital problems. Short-term couple's counseling and a support group were recommended to help with communication and emotional isolation. The integrated support of the medical and counseling staff could help the R.'s through this crisis with a renewed sense of self-esteem and control.

SUMMARY

Infertility is a life crisis impacting on all aspects of a couple's life. The medical evaluation, diagnosis, and treatment for infertility takes at least several months and can extend over a period of years. Throughout this stressful period, couples struggle with a range of emotions which include anxiety, sadness, guilt, anger, loss of self-esteem and hopelessness. Without the opportunity to acknowledge and understand these feelings, couples may experience deterioration in marital and interpersonal relationships, job functioning, and overall health and well-being.

A psychosocial evaluation of the infertile couple can be an important tool to the attending physician. Frequently, new information is obtained that may be important to treatment or clinical insights useful in dealing with the patient. It can also serve as a lifeline to the infertile couple, who often feels defective and isolated. The interview provides the couple with the opportunity to ventilate feelings and receive information on coping with the stress, thus preventing future problems. The couple feels respected, responded to, more normal, and less isolated. Further, a relationship with the social worker has been established which aids in the transition to ongoing counseling if needed. The social worker, acting as a communication link between patient and medical staff, has the opportunity to act as an advocate for both parties. The psychosocial evaluation can be one of the many challenges and opportunities that exist for social workers in reproductive medicine.

REFERENCES

Batterman, R. (1985). Comprehensive approach to treating infertility. *Health and Social Work*, *10*(1), 46-54.
Berger, D. (1977). The role of the psychiatrist in a reproductive biology clinic. *Fertility and Sterility*, *28*(2), 141-145.
Bresnick, E. (1981). A holistic approach to the treatment of the crisis of infertility. *Journal of Marital and Family Therapy*, 181-188.
Bresnick, E. & Taymor, M. (1979). The role of counseling in infertility. *Fertility and Sterility*, *32*(2), 181-188.

Christie, G. L. (1980). The psychological and social management of the infertile couple. In R. J. Pepperell, B. Hudson & C. Wood (Eds.), *The Infertile Couple*. Edinburgh and New York: Churchill Livingstone, 229-247.

Cooper, B., Harwin, B. G., Delpa, C. & Sheperd, M. (1975). Mental health care in the community: An evaluative study. *Psychological Medicine*, *5*(4), 372-380.

Ellsworth, L. & Shain, R. (1985). Psychosocial and psychophysiologic aspects of reproduction: The need for improved study design. *Fertility and Sterility*, *44*(4), 449-452.

Fein, D. (1985). Psychotherapy for infertility. *Fertility and Sterility*, *44*(6), 855-856.

Keye, W. R., Jr. (1984). Psychosexual responses to infertility. *Clinical Obstetrics and Gynecology*, *27*(3), 760-766.

Kraft, A., Palombo, J., Mitchell, D., Dean, C., Meyers, S. & Schmidt, A. (1980). The psychological dimensions of infertility. *American Journal of Orthopsychiatry*, *50*(4), 618-628.

Linderman, E. (1965). Sympotomology and management of acute grief. In H. J. Pared (Ed.), *Crisis Intervention: Selected Readings*. New York: Family Service Association of America, 7-21.

Mahlstedt, P. (1980). The psychological component of infertility. *Fertility and Sterility*, *43*(3), 335-346.

Mazor, M. (1979). Barren couples. *Psychology Today*, 22, 101-112.

Mechnic, D. (1980). The management of psychosocial problems in primary medical care: A potential role for social work. *Journal of Human Stress*, *6*(4), 16-21.

Menning, B. (1977). *Infertility*. Englewood Cliffs, NJ: Prentice-Hall, Inc.

Menning, B. (1975). The infertile couple: A plea for advocacy. *Child Welfare*, *54*, 454-460.

Menning, B. (1980). The emotional needs of infertile couples. *Fertility and Sterility*, *34*(4),313-319.

Rapoport, L. (1962). The state of crisis: Some theoretical considerations. *Social Service Review*, *36*, 211-217.

Seibel, M. & Taymor, M. (1982). Emotional aspects of infertility. *Fertility and Sterility*, *37*, 137-145.

Shapiro, C. H. (1982). The impact of infertility on the marital relationship. *Social Casework: The Journal of Contemporary Social Work*, *63*, 387-393.

Sorrel, P. & DeCherney, A. (1985). Psychotherapeutic intervention for treatment of couples with secondary infertility. *Fertility and Sterility*, *43*(6), 897-900.

Staff. (1986). Emergence of medical psychotherapy: The new role of the mental health practitioner in the health care system (Part II). *Medical Psychotherapist*, *2*(1), 1-2.

Coping with Infertility

Jeanne Fleming
Kenneth Burry

SUMMARY. Individuals experiencing infertility have described their pain as grief. Results of an exploratory survey indicate that persons experiencing infertility use a variety of techniques to cope with their feelings. The authors suggest that infertility grief should be viewed as a process which may require the mastery of ongoing coping strategies and support.

Approximately 15-20% of all married couples in the United States are infertile (Kraft et al., 1980). These couples are generally young and otherwise healthy people who may have had little experience with the health care system. Appropriate diagnosis and treatment of infertility may take six months to a year or more. Treatment of infertility may quickly result in a successful pregnancy. In many other situations, however, infertile couples spend years trying to build a family with uncertain outcome. An eventual successful pregnancy occurs in only about 50% of the cases despite years of medical treatment of infertility (Menning, 1977).

A wide variety of emotional and behavioral responses to the infertility experience have been described in the literature. Reactions include symptoms of crisis (Bresnick, 1981), depression and mourning (Shapiro, 1982), anxiety (Berger, 1980), and feelings of sadness, anger, confusion, desperation, hurt, fear, embarrassment, humiliation, disappointment, unfairness, and unfulfillment. Behavioral reactions such as disorganization, distractibility, exhaustion, fatigue moodiness, unpredictability and obsessive thoughts were also attributed to the psychological impact of the infertility experience (Valentine, 1986). Menning (1977) refers to the "grief" of infertility.

A variety of factors may contribute to the emotional impact of the infertility experience. Infertility and lengthy medical treatment delays the couple's goal of birthing and parenting a child. A major life goal is thwarted. Messages about the importance of biological family building are pervasive in our society. An assumption of fertility and the mandate to reproduce is internalized to the extent that some individuals experiencing infertility feel like failures. Clinical evidence suggests that when diagnosis and treatment of a medical condition is prolonged, emotions fluctuate along with their medical condition and treatment, a possible additional stressor for the infertile couple (Johnston, 1984). Additional factors contributing to the ease or difficulty with which an individual responds to his or her infertility includes: the importance to each person and the couple of a biological child; felt pressure from extended family or friends to have a baby; and/or the degree to which supportive social connections are available (Clapp, 1985; Hinton, 1981; Mahlstedt, 1985; Siebel et al., 1982).

In what ways do persons experiencing infertility cope with their feelings? The results of an exploratory survey of 83 participants who volunteered to complete a questionnaire of open-ended questions are discussed.

DATA COLLECTION

The investigators of this exploratory survey solicited volunteers from Resolve, Inc., a national, nonprofit organization which offers counseling, referral, and support to people with problems of infertility. A request for volunteers willing to participate in research on the emotional impact of infertility was published in national and chapter newsletters in 1984. Eighty-three completed questionnaires were returned.

The questionnaire consisted of closed and open-ended questions designed to provide a beginning understanding of persons experiencing infertility. Of the 83 subjects participating in the project, 70 were female and 13 were male. The age of participants ranged from 25 to 41-years-old.

DISCUSSION

Consistent with previously described research on the psychological impact of infertility, feelings of sadness, anger, frustration, inferiority, loneliness, guilt, and fear were reported by persons experiencing infertility who responded to the survey. In contrast, feelings of hopefulness, contentment, and love for spouse were also reported. Participants reported the use of a variety of coping strategies. The choices participants made regarding their family-building included: adoption, child-free living, and/or a successful past or current pregnancy. The majority of those surveyed, however, indicated that a decision or final plan had not been made regarding the future of their family. Most of the subjects indicated that the prolonged length of time that infertility was experienced influenced their emotional functioning. Some respondents indicated experiencing a loss of hope while others felt it became easier to cope with their infertility over time. The majority of persons responding indicated that the experience of infertility affected their marriage. Many reported that infertility strained their relationship, but an equal number reported a closer, more open relationship.

Respondents described *avoidance* of various situations in their efforts to cope with infertility. Contact with pregnant women, contact with children, and child-oriented events were identified as frequently avoided situations. The strategy of *distraction* from infertility was also described by participants as a way of managing feelings pertaining to infertility. These included taking trips or increasing participation in activities, class, or work.

When asked whether feelings about infertility were resolved, the majority of respondents indicated that they were *not* resolved. Many of the participants felt that development of long-range plans to cope and adjust to their infertility helped, but they indicated that the pain of infertility would never subside.

When referring to loss and grief, Schneider (1984) defines resolution as:

> acknowledging in a shared way that what is past is over; that it has both positive and negative aspects; that the bereaved contributed to the loss and that there were no limits to the contri-

bution he or she made; and that, finally, the person discovered some way to make restitution for contributions either to the loss or for the way in which it was grieved. (p. 194)

Responses by participants in this study suggest that "resolution" may be neither an appropriate term nor an appropriate goal for the loss of fertility. The experience of infertility may not lend itself to putting the past behind. Perhaps, the ongoing process of coping describes the experience of infertility more accurately. Hinsie and Campbell (1970) define coping as:

adjusting; adapting; successfully meeting a challenge. Coping mechanisms are all the ways, both conscious and unconscious, which a person uses in adjusting to environmental demands without altering his [sic] goals or purposes. (p. 163)

Survey responses suggest that coping mechanisms such as distraction and avoidance seem to be a common method for dealing with the ongoing experience of infertility. Infertility does not appear to be experienced as a single, identifiable event which can be resolved and then forgotten. Throughout the life cycle, persons experience reminders of their infertility, for example, during the application and process of adoption, or during times when cohorts are celebrating their children's graduation, marriage, or grandparenthood. In this regard, response to infertility may be more like one's response to a chronic illness (requiring coping strategies for adaptation and adjustment over time) than a response to an acute illness (requiring resolution).

The implications of this exploratory study suggest that persons experiencing infertility may benefit from learning to cope with infertility as others learn to cope with chronic illnesses or chronic emotional dilemmas. If people can be provided with information which realistically portrays their situation and taught methods useful in differentiating and handling difficult issues, they may be more likely to feel productive and proud that they have learned new skills in handling life's challenges. For persons experiencing infertility, ongoing support, and counseling throughout the life cycle may be much more appropriate than immediate first-aid or crisis intervention. As was remarked by one respondent:

Infertility is like a broken bone, when it heals, it will be stronger than ever, but on rainy days it hurts. . . . You may not be proud of breaking your bone, but you can be proud you developed stronger muscles using crutches.

REFERENCES

Berger, D. (1977). The role of the psychiatrist in a reproductive biology clinic. *Fertility and Sterility, 28*(2), 141-145.

Bresnick, E. (1981). A holistic approach to the treatment of the crisis of infertility. *Journal of Marital and Family Therapy*, 181-188.

Clapp, D. (1985). Emotional responses to infertility: Nursing interventions. *Journal of Gynecological & Neonatal Nursing Supplement, 32.*

Hinsie, Leland & Campbell, R.J. (1970). *Psychiatric dictionary.* New York: Oxford University Press.

Hinton, M. (1981, April). The stress of infertility and how to cope. *Resolve Newsletter,* p. 7.

Johnston, P. (1984). *An adopter's advocate.* Fort Wayne, IN: Perspectives Press, 16-52.

Kraft, A. D. & Polombo, J. et al. (1980). The psychological dimensions of infertility. *American Journal of Orthopsychiatry, 50*(4), 618-628.

Mahlstedt, P. (1985). The psychological component of infertility. *Fertility & Sterility, 43*(3), 335-346.

Menning, B. (1977). *A guide for the childless couple.* New Jersey: Prentice-Hall, Inc., 3-163.

Schneider, John. (1984). *Stress, Loss & Grief.* Baltimore: University Park Press.

Seibel, M., Seibel, M. & Taymor, L. (1982). Emotional aspects of infertility. *Fertility & Sterility, 37*(2), 137-145.

Shapiro, C.H. (1982). The impact of infertility on the marital relationship. *Social Casework, 63,* 387-393.

Valentine, Deborah. (1986). Psychological impact of infertility: Identifying issues and needs. *Social Work in Health Care, 11*(4), 61-69.

Reproductive Losses and Grieving

Patricia Conway
Deborah Valentine

SUMMARY. This article presents the findings from a qualitative research study exploring ten couples' experiences with reproductive loss, infertility, miscarriage, and stillbirth. Following the primary loss, that of a biological child, couples identified five categories of associated losses: the experience of pregnancy, childbirth and breastfeeding; parenting; control; relationships; and one's view of oneself as a fertile individual. Feelings of shock, unfairness, fear, anger, a sense of being different from others, and intense sadness characterized the grieving process. Six factors mediated the grieving process: multiple losses, existing relationships, one's perception of being the victim or "cause" of the loss, gender, recognition of the loss, and cultural factors. The quality of grieving did change over time, but the impact of reproductive loss never completely disappeared.

Events in our past comprise our history and directly impact the rest of our lives. In addition, current events trigger new feelings about old experiences. One physically healthy and professionally successful woman fainted unexpectedly and without apparent cause. When trying to piece together the events of the day, she realized that that particular day was the due date of her "hoped for child" who had miscarried seven months earlier. Another woman, as a result of a new job in a hospice setting, became intimately involved with people working through their own or a loved one's impending death. She subsequently experienced new grieving for her child who had died in stillbirth ten years previously. Putting past experiences in perspective allows us to continue functioning and to enjoy life, but it in no way erases the impact of those experiences.

How might these and other reproductive loss experiences be viewed as normative so that isolated incidents "make sense" in the context of one's whole life? In an effort to better understand the answers to this question, this article presents the findings from a qualitative research study which explored couples' experiences with reproductive loss. The framework for the exploration and analysis of these experiences was constructed from a review of the literature on loss and grief in general as well as the literature specific to reproductive loss. The following discussion focuses on the nature of these losses, the grieving process following reproductive loss, and factors mediating the grieving process.

REPRODUCTIVE LOSS: A REVIEW OF THE LITERATURE

The Nature of Reproductive Loss

Reproductive losses identified in the literature are infertility, miscarriage, and stillbirth. Infertility is routinely defined as a condition in which "a successful pregnancy, leading to a live birth, has not occurred within a year of regular sexual relations without contraception" (Mazor & Simons, 1984, p. xvi). Although this term theoretically includes both miscarriage, the loss of the fetus between conception and five months of age, and stillbirth, "death before birth of a fetus that is at least 20 weeks of gestation" (Borg & Lasker, 1981, p. 242), infertility literature frequently focuses on the inability to conceive. The term pregnancy loss is used in some cases to mean miscarriage or stillbirth (Friedman & Gradstein, 1982; Herz, 1984). Reproductive loss will be used in this paper as a more comprehensive term to include the inability to conceive and the death of a fetus before birth.

The primary loss from infertility, miscarriage, or stillbirth is obviously that of a biological child. As with any loss, however, this leads to many associated losses, including:

1. lost fantasies;
2. the loss of genetic continuity;
3. loss of one's self-image as a fertile person;

4. the loss of the successful pregnancy and birth experience;
5. loss of the experience of breastfeeding;
6. loss of the opportunity to move to the next stage in the family life cycle;
7. relationship losses;
8. loss of the parenting experience; and
9. losses for other family members such as potential grandparents (Herz, 1984; Klaus & Kennel, 1976; Knapp & Peppers, 1980; Menning, 1977; Menning, 1980).

The Grieving Process Following Reproductive Loss

The grieving process following reproductive loss as identified by different theorists varies in terms of the words used, but all include three general phases of emotions and behaviors: (1) the initial awareness, characterized by shock and denial; (2) a "deep grieving" stage of intense sadness and anger; and (3) a final phase of "adaptation" to the loss (Bowlby, 1980; Mazor, 1984; Menning, 1980; Schneider, 1984; Silverman, 1981). The term "phase" is used as opposed to "stage" to indicate that there is no set order to the phases and that movement between phases is very fluid (Schneider, 1984). Viewing the phases of grieving as flexible seems particularly appropriate for reproductive loss, which usually encompasses multiple losses over time.

Although return of energy, a sense of humor, looking to the future, and relief are identified as characteristics of the "adaptation" or "resolution" phase of grieving, differences of opinion exist about whether grieving is ever resolved and ended (Kirkley-Best & Kellner, 1982; Menning, 1980; Peppers & Knapp, 1980). Menning (1980) states that "feelings are never laid away forever; they may be activated by special reminders, such as anniversaries of losses, or by new and different crises" (p. 317). Peppers and Knapp (1980) write that the "grieving comes to a close" for persons able to reach this adaptation phase of grieving. They do, however, note that frequently a "shadow grief" remains, "'something'. . . difficult to pinpoint exactly; but because of it their lives will never be the same again" (p. 47). The words of one woman poignantly illustrate this shadow grief:

It doesn't matter now to anyone.
No one ever knew.
But now and then,
    Along the day,
I look at first graders
With their Snoopy lunchboxes
And tender paintings of trees and frogs,
And I think about those first feelings
    of movement
    and growth.
                            (Malloy, 1975, p.70)

Feelings identified with the grieving process include guilt, shame, envy, anger, helplessness or lack of control, sadness or grief, surprise, denial and isolation (Herz, 1984; Menning, 1980; Raphael, 1983). "Without question, (though,) the most compelling feeling . . . is grief" (Menning, 1980, p. 316).

Factors Mediating the Grieving Process

The timing, intensity, and content of the grieving process may vary. In general, the following factors mediate grieving: age, type of loss and type of attachment, number of losses, existing relationships, pre-loss personality, whether the person grieving perceives him or herself as a victim or initiator of the loss, and whether or not the loss is recognized (Schneider, 1984). Another potential mediating factor specifically related to reproductive loss is gender (Berezin, 1982).

Age

Especially for women, age is a critical childbearing factor. The rates for both infertility and miscarriages increase with a woman's age (Adler, 1986; Menning, 1977). "Even more dramatically, the rate of anxiety goes up as the number of years in which to conceive again shrinks" (Adler, 1986, p. 66).

Age might also influence the grieving process with respect to miscarriages and stillbirth. "Out of time" losses, when persons die "before their time," are particularly powerful losses. Couples expect to conceive and bear live children, not to experience the death of their "hoped for" child (Palmer & Noble, 1986; Stringham, Riley & Ross, 1982, p. 326). Schneider (1984) suggests that these "out of time" losses frequently result in more complex grieving.

Type of Loss

The type of loss, i.e., inability to conceive, miscarriage, or still-birth, may result in a different quality or process of grieving. Couples who have never been pregnant may grieve a different loss than those who experience a loss during a pregnancy.

The time during the pregnancy when the loss occurred might also influence the grieving process if parents bond differently to a fetus at varying times during the pregnancy. Klaus and Kennell (1976) suggest that there is a "sensitive period" immediately following birth when men and women attach to their child (p. 50). What bonding occurs before birth that would lead to grieving if the fetus was lost? Klaus and Kennell (1976) identify two stages of pregnancy for the woman: (1) acceptance of the pregnancy, with the fetus seen as part of herself, and (2) perception of the fetus as a separate individual, beginning with quickening. For the man, attachment may occur differently and more slowly because he does not have a physical relationship with the fetus (Peppers & Knapp, 1980). This indicates that women may grieve differently depending on whether the loss occurred during the first or second stage. Also, men may grieve differently than women because bonding to the fetus occurs on a different time schedule.

Interestingly, Peppers and Knapp (1980) found no difference in feelings experienced (sadness, insomnia, guilt feelings) by women who had suffered miscarriage and those who had suffered either a stillbirth or a neonatal death. They did find that emotions varied in intensity by the type of loss. Women experiencing miscarriages felt more guilt and those experiencing stillbirth felt more bitterness. In fact, the grieving process following miscarriage and stillbirth looks like the grieving process after the loss of a long-time close family member (Klaus & Kennell, 1976).

Number of Losses

The number of losses experienced by couples desiring to parent may also influence the grief experience. An individual's capacity to grieve is limited (Friedman & Gradstein, 1982; Schneider, 1984). Among couples with reproductive difficulties, the potential losses are multiple, i.e., difficult conception, miscarriage, stillbirth, loss of friends, and financial loss.

Existing Relationships

Existing relationships between a husband and wife and between a couple and others may mediate the grieving process following reproductive loss. The quality of the marital relationship prior to the loss seems particularly important for couples experiencing reproductive loss. Infertility, miscarriage, and stillbirth places special strains on the relationship (Friedman & Gradstein, 1982; Shapiro, 1982). "The strength of the relationship prior to bereavement, and what each partner is able to bring into the situation in the form of earlier experiences in dealing with frustration and defeat, heavily influence the denouement" (Berezin, 1982, p. 34). Bierkens (1975) noted that the bulk of the 180 persons in his study who were childless listed their spouse as the greatest source of support.

Relationships with family members, friends, and the medical community also play a role in mediating the grief process. Unfortunately, external support is frequently absent (Herz, 1984; Hertz, 1982; Menning, 1980; Raphael, 1983; Schwartz, 1984). Bierkens (1975) found that childless couples experienced continual discomfort as other family members had children. The discomfort increased when families with children did not talk with childless couples about their pain.

Pre-Loss Personality

The personality of the individual prior to loss most likely influences the grieving process. Kraft, Palombo, Mitchell, Dean, Meyers, and Schmidt (1980) found that "those with a positive, integrated sense of self, . . . relatively nontraumatic childhoods, . . . (and) with strong, caring, protective parents" (p. 624) were able to adapt successfully to the tasks presented as a result of reproductive loss. Caution must be employed, however, when examining pre-loss personality and making a determination about how it impacts on grieving after infertility, miscarriage, or stillbirth.

Couples are routinely seen following a loss, not prior to that loss. A body of literature has developed about the personality of couples who are infertile, taking the post-loss characteristics of infertile couples and defining those characteristics as the cause of the loss (Herz, 1984). One must be cautious about assuming that current characteristics are causal and preexisting when in fact they might be consequences of the loss.

Initiator vs. Victim of Loss

A particularly sensitive topic for couples experiencing reproductive loss is their perception of what, and therefore, who, "causes" the loss. Couples search for a "cause" for their loss, and may blame themselves, their spouse, and/or the medical profession (Raphael, 1983). Feelings vary from guilt to anger depending on one's perception of the cause of the loss.

Loss Recognition

Schneider (1984) indicates that grieving is more complicated when a loss is not recognized as having occurred. Reproductive losses, "quiet tragedies," may be invisible to outsiders (Ilse & Burns, 1985; Kirkley-Best & Kellner, 1982, p. 420; Menning, 1980; Raphael, 1983; Stack, 1980; Stack, 1984) and may not be fully acknowledged by the couple experiencing the loss. Even the death of a child during birth is frequently dismissed by outsiders because the family has not had time to get to know that child.

> The death of a stillborn baby, as in any loss, requires a period of grieving, but because the baby is seen as a "nonperson" and is largely unacknowledged by society, families are often left unsupported in their grief. (Stringham, Riley & Ross, 1982, p. 322)

Gender

The literature suggests that men and women respond differently to pregnancy loss (Berezin, 1982; Brand, 1982). This may occur because of the differing biological roles for men and women during pregnancy, as discussed in a previous section.

> In the earliest months of the pregnancy the mother's attachment to the developing baby is usually intense, for the baby is harbored and nurtured by her body. The father's attachment is less intense, for the unborn baby is less real to him, and he knows it only through fantasy and identification with the mother. (Raphael, 1983, p. 230)

Silverman (1981) argues men and women are socialized differently and therefore experience the same loss differently. Because women's roles involving relationships are primary for them, losses involving relationships will result in greater grieving for women than men.

> If indeed a woman's sense of self is inextricably linked with her attachments and affiliations, it is clearly not possible for her to suffer a loss or rupture in an attachment without feeling that her very identity has been fundamentally damaged. (p. 22)

Also, grieving could be experienced differently because men are socialized to "be strong" and women are to "be emotional." A husband's response to grieving a miscarriage might be action-oriented, at a time when his wife needs to talk repeatedly about the loss (Herz, 1984). A rift between the husband and wife experiencing reproductive loss may occur because their response to grief differs.

METHODOLOGY

To further explore reproductive loss, associated losses, and the resulting grieving process, ten couples were asked to share their experiences related to reproductive loss. These couples, recruited through public announcements and word of mouth, were all married, and ranged in age from 25 to 37. All the couples but one were Caucasian and all but one had an associate of arts degree or higher. Four of the couples had never conceived; five experienced miscarriages; one couple had a child following five years of infertility and were again pregnant at the time of the interview. Another couple, infertile for many years, experienced a Caesarean birth. Two of the couples had adopted—one a child from another country and another, four children. A variety of medical problems associated with infertility were reported, including low sperm count, sperm antibodies, endometriosis, scar tissue, and tubal pregnancy.

Each couple was interviewed in their home or business for approximately two hours, with both husband and wife present. The interviews were taped, guided by a semistructured schedule developed from the preceding literature review. Basic demographic information was gathered and general questions were asked to explore the history of the reproductive loss experience. Information about feelings, supports and nonsupports, and the decision-making process around parenting decisions were also obtained. (The interview schedule is available upon request.)

Each of the tapes was then transcribed and compared. The general literature on loss and grieving and literature specific to reproductive loss provide the categories for analysis:

1. associated losses;
2. feelings experienced during the grieving process; and
3. factors mediating the grieving process.

COUPLES' EXPERIENCE
WITH REPRODUCTIVE LOSS:
A QUALITATIVE ANALYSIS

Reproductive Losses Experienced

At the heart of reproductive loss is the loss of a child. Couples wishing to parent report intense sadness when they are unable to share their lives with a child or carry their family into the next generation. In the words of one woman participating in the research, "I just wanted to have a baby really really bad." Other losses identified in this study include the loss of pregnancy and parenthood, loss of control over one's life, loss of relationships, and loss of one's view of oneself as a "fertile" individual.

Loss of the Experience of Pregnancy, Childbirth, and Breastfeeding

Women who had never been pregnant stated that they missed both the social and the biological experience of pregnancy. Women consistently reported that they were excluded from conversations with friends about the pregnancy experience. "I couldn't talk to my friends anymore because I wasn't part of them." "Two good friends were pregnant at the same time and delivered at the same time. It hit me when I visited them in the hospital. I felt left out of what they were talking about. I don't and never will have the experience of labor." Husbands suggested that their wives experienced sadness about reproductive loss differently than they, "With ladies, it's the first thing you talk about. You talk about your children." "It didn't bother me as much as my wife because guys aren't around children and mothers and females talking about children and pregnancy and all that. It's not as big a problem for guys."

Women concurred. "I have to deal with more than my husband; I miss not wearing maternity clothes." Although on the surface the comment about wearing maternity clothes appears superficial, it came up consistently. The concern about maternity clothes seems to represent several other losses. Maternity clothes signify publicly that a woman is experiencing a change in status; frequently this "special time" signifies a move from childhood to adulthood. Also, buying special clothes for a special time provides nurturing for a women who is preparing to nurture another.

Women also miss the biological experience of pregnancy. One woman described this as the "glow of pregnancy," a special time biologically. "I must give up my dream. I really want the pregnancy experience." Another woman who experienced infertility for several years and then parented through adoption of four children and birth of a son through Caesarean birth expressed sadness because she missed a natural childbirth. Additionally, women who wish to breastfeed lose that experience.

Loss of Parenting

Losses associated with parenthood include loss of the parenting role, loss of generativity, and loss of moving to the next stage in the family life cycle. One woman stated that she had to change her view of herself as a mother to that of a career woman. Another couple had waited to parent until the husband was out of school and had a stable job. The wife quit work to be at home and mother. Now they face the prospect of a childfree future. "All my life, I have wanted to be a mother and I wanted that to be the focal point of my life. When you have that taken away from you, you really have to decide what you are going to do with the rest of your life — when you don't have that opportunity to parent."

Men also lose their role as parent. One woman described her husband as "having a flair with children. He would make a good father." Another father declared that he would be like anyone else if he had children, taking them to baseball games and pageants!

The loss of generativity includes the loss of family genetic continuity, of family traditions, and of one's own continuity. As one couple put it, "It is fun to satisfy the curiosity about what one's own child would look like, that the child has it's father's nose."

Families experiencing reproductive loss miss moving to the next stage of the family life cycle (successful pregnancy and parenthood). "Marriage is in stages. We wanted to move to the next stage." "You're not right with the world. You're different because you have not been able to follow the pattern of life that everyone doesn't think about following." "I had this sense of continuity and the continuity was chopped off."

Loss of Control

In all ten cases, loss of control was mentioned as an important factor. "This is the first time in my life I have not had control over it." Men and women experience a lack of control over their reproductive capacities. Couples mentioned that their previous efforts to prevent pregnancy and thus control their fertility were for naught. "Now we laugh about all those years I took the pill. What a waste!"

Couples experiencing reproductive loss are constantly vulnerable to intrusions by staff in the medical profession and adoption agencies. "When you go to the infertility specialist, you have to bare every aspect of your intimate relationship. You have to get naked in front of all of these doctors and all of these nurses. You have to . . . I couldn't tell you the number of people I've had to take my clothes off for. And being approved for adoption is sort of baring yourself like that too."

Relationship Losses

Couples experiencing reproductive losses face a threat to their marital relationship. The loss of common dreams and the need to reassess those dreams are experienced. Furthermore, the complications resulting from the artificial intrusion into their relationship by medical personnel, adoption workers, and counselors is an additional loss of privacy. Infertility "tears us apart because our life is laid out."

One couple, when asked how they felt when they did not get pregnant, responded, "It was awful. The pressure every time you had sex; it was the only thing you thought about." Reproductive losses are a direct assault on the sexual relationship of couples. Impotence was a common reaction to the stress. "It would have eased our minds if some doctor had said this might happen. The wife then thinks she is undesirable."

Women may react to the pressures by avoiding intercourse in order to avoid the worries about whether pregnancy will occur. "There was a little bit of — if I don't have sex when I ovulate, I can't possibly be pregnant; then I don't have to worry about whether I will menstruate. Next, I avoid sex altogether to get relief from wondering if I'm pregnant."

The View of Oneself as a Fertile Individual

Men and women unable to conceive stressed the loss of self-esteem that results from being labeled "infertile." One man who was infertile described men with infertility problems as "wimps." Another negatively responded to the suggestion of donor insemination because it was like "bringing in the A Team." The loss of fertility was frequently described by women as a physical loss. "I felt like I had cancer." "It's like a death or deformity. People don't want to be close to it." "It's a scar."

Grieving Following Reproductive Loss

Couples indicated that their grieving changed over time in intensity, but there appeared to be no consensus about the length of time the process, including initial awareness, deep grieving, and adaptation, takes. "It hurts, but the hurt fades." One woman stated that in the early stages of learning about the couple's infertility, she "thought about infertility every day, all day, for almost a year." Another said, "I keep thinking that one day, we would reach an acceptance, because every day I feel a little bit different, but it's been three years now and I still hope that one day I will wake up and understand. But I might be 50!" After several year's experience with infertility, one woman stated, "It's just a big loss. And it still hurts. And it always will."

The grieving process was also influenced by the recurring losses characteristic of infertility, miscarriage, and stillbirth and by the lack of a clear time when a loss occurred. Medical treatment for infertility and prevention of miscarriages and stillbirths frequently continues for years. One couple noted that the five years they spent going through medical interventions was tough. The wife reached the "pits of depression" after three years when she began to acknowledge that they really might not be able to conceive. Her husband, though, stated that "if people want children badly enough, they will go to any extreme to try to get them." Couples also experienced an "emotional roller coaster" for years, with sadness and depression at each menstruation.

The inability to identify a crisis point when one can acknowledge the occurrence of a loss occurred may make the progress through grieving seem immeasurably slow. One couple who had no clear medical message about whether they would ever conceive said it took them "six months to one year to get to the 'might as well move on' stage.'' Other couples stated that they almost wished the doctor would give them a stopping place, telling them that fertility would never be a possibility so they could move on. Some couples made their own decision to stop the endless medical interventions. ''When we decided we had done everything we could about infertility, we decided to adopt. We had to decide; do we want children (biologically) or a family? It was more damaging to us as a couple to continue the infertility study.''

Feelings Experienced by Couples During the Grieving Process

Six feelings characteristic of the grieving process were identified by couples: shock, unfairness and envy, fear, anger, feeling different, and grief or hurt.

Shock. A woman reported feeling like she felt pregnant for two weeks following a miscarriage. Another stated, ''When the doctor said, 'You have to face it. You may never get pregnant,' my first reaction was panic. I wanted to slap him. I thought, oh, no! I can't! Even if I never get pregnant, . . . I don't *think* I could ever . . . I don't know. I didn't believe him at that point. I wasn't ready. And I still don't believe him. He said I had endometriosis and I said, 'I do not!' ''

Unfairness, envy, being cheated. ''It's like watching other people with a lollipop and you can't have one. You're jealous.'' ''We want a child. We've got a lot to offer . . . You go out and you see so and so with a child. At first, when I found out that I couldn't . . . that I had a low sperm count . . . you don't mean to, but there's a hate. At church, you see children, you start feeling bad, just want to walk away.''

Fear. ''It's scary to look at a woman in her 40s who wanted to have children but couldn't.'' One woman stated she felt fear and panic, a ''desperate feeling that has gotten worse, and that fear is intensified by my age.''

Anger. Couples expressed anger repeatedly, at each other, their families and friends, other couples with children, a culture that values parenting, the adoption process, and the medical profession. ''I'm angry in general; it doesn't seem fair!'' ''My husband handled

the miscarriage badly. He was not supportive, doting, consoling."
"All my friends had kids. At my lowest point, I resented everything." A couple choosing to be childfree were angry with Resolve,
a national support group for persons who are infertile, stating "they
see parenting as the only solution."

Feeling different from others. "We didn't have anyone going
through the same problems." "I feel different because I don't have
a baby and we are not going to adopt."

Grief, hurt, unhappiness, a nightmare. Deep hurt characterized
all the couples' experiences. A male, when told his sperm count
was too low to allow conception, felt "kind of like a stump inside.
That was my hardest step." Another stated, "I grieved like a child
had died. The baby I never had was dead." "It (the miscarriage)
hurt and knowing that there was nothing to reward you in the end
hurt even more. Two weeks later I was putting up my small children's clothes and became hysterical, crying for at least an hour."

Factors Mediating the Grieving Process

Factors mediating the grieving process identified in the literature
and supported by the comments of the ten couples interviewed included: number of losses, existing relationships, whether the person
grieving perceived him or herself to be a victim or the initiator of
the loss, whether the loss is recognized or not, and gender. An
additional mediating factor, culture, emerged from the couple's
comments. The small sample does not allow a comparison of age,
type of loss, or pre-loss personality, which are other potential mediating factors suggested by Schneider (1984).

Number of Losses

Multiple losses seemed to increase the intensity of grieving and
to prolong the grieving process. One couple experienced infertility,
adoption, and childbirth. Their "resolution" of the pain of infertility was reawakened when they lost a child through miscarriage and
subsequently were infertile. Even though the family now includes
five children, the mother said, "I am disappointed every month
when I am not pregnant."

When reproductive losses occurred simultaneously with the death of a parent, intense sadness prevailed. A woman whose father had died nine months previously felt overwhelmed by his death. She experienced not only sadness, but also increased responsibility for her mother at a time when she needed additional support for her own reproductive loss. "My father died in January. That just compounded it (sadness following miscarriage). I just didn't think about it, I just grieved for my father. Then for a while I thought I was just going to burst. There was just so much pain."

Existing Relationships

Couples mentioned existing relationships with each other, their family and friends, and the medical community as important factors in their grieving process. Most frequently, couples stated that their primary support during grieving was each other. One couple, though, appeared very sad that their reproductive loss experiences had not brought them closer together.

Friends were viewed as nonsupportive usually, probably due to their feelings of discomfort. For instance, two couples mentioned that friends were afraid to discuss their pregnancy with the couple experiencing reproductive loss. Friends' responses seemed to influence the couples' grieving pattern by suppressing the couples' ability to recognize and talk about their loss. One man stated that he could not tell his golf buddies that he was missing their usual Thursday evening golf to complete the research interview. Another couple was told by friends that they should not feel so bad about their infertility and subsequent miscarriage because "at lease they were able to get pregnant."

The inability of families to discuss reproductive loss was pervasive. "Mother won't discuss it as a problem. She says, 'you worry too much. Everything's going to be fine.' I don't think she can. Don't think she knows what to say. I think that's what's wrong with our family."

Family members may be unable to be supportive because they are experiencing their own related loss. "What about our parents, they will never have grandkids." Also, lack of support may result from discomfort family members experience with other family members' fertility. "My sister is pregnant now and now we are apologizing for that." A couple going through in vitro fertilization (ultimately unsuccessful) stated their parents found themselves in a difficult position. A sister became pregnant at the same time, and the parents were expected to be excited about one child's pregnancy without distressing their other child experiencing infertility.

Finally, lack of understanding by family members was common. One man's brother-in-law recommended that the infertile man "eat more oysters." Another common but unhelpful recommendation by family members was "relax."

Unfortunately, the helping profession did not facilitate the grieving process in most cases. The nurse chatting about her children throughout one woman's extensive and painful infertility tests enhanced the infertile woman's sadness about her lack of children. Women hospitalized for infertility tests, artificial insemination, and miscarriage were routinely placed on obstetrical wards with excited couples enjoying their infants. Doctors who said, "Get a bottle of wine and go to the beach for the weekend" or "Smoke a cigarette, drink some wine, and relax" increased a couple's sense of failure and personal responsibility for that failure. The medical profession also frequently did not attend to associated losses that might appropriately have been softened by professional assistance. "None of the doctors ever asked about how the infertility affected our sex life."

When medical professionals were perceived as supportive, though, unpleasant feelings were decreased. One woman credited a thoughtful nurse for making her stay on an obstetrics ward less painful. The nurse stayed with her during night time feedings, a particularly poignant period for the woman.

Perceived Status as Initiator vs. Victim of Loss

Each person experiencing reproductive loss may grieve differently based on his or her perception of their own role in "causing" the loss. Couples always talked about where the blocks to reproduction occurred, which meant they talked about their perception of their own and their partner's role in the reproductive loss. For couples unable to conceive, support for each other appeared critical.

When a man with a low sperm count mentioned "my problem," his wife interjected "our problem." Women said: "It's not just one party's responsibility. I couldn't have come to terms with it (infertility from endometriosis) if he wasn't helping me." "Never once did he say it's my fault." "No one blamed anyone. He never ever made me feel like it was my fault. I remember saying, 'I bet you wished you married your old girlfriend. Don't you feel cheated?'" In the one case where a spouse appeared angry because the partner was infertile, sadness pervaded the entire interview.

Gender

Gender did appear to mediate the grieving process; couples insisted that the husband's grieving was different than the wife's. "I like to talk about things, my husband would say put it to rest" was the common sentiment. "I knew I had this problem that he did not want to hear about. I just wanted to have a baby really really bad. I've always wanted kids. I love children. To be told all this and to realize what it meant, it was a real shock. It took a long time to absorb what it meant, all the dreams, . . . kind of out the window." After a woman remarked that the hardest time for her was when her husband would not talk about the infertility or miscarriage, her husband stated simply, "I just didn't want to talk about it."

Not only did men and women express their grieving differently, but they seemed to experience a different level of intensity of grieving. As stated previously in the section, "Loss of the Experience of Pregnancy," women and men both thought that women were sadder and had to make more adjustments than men.

Loss Recognition

Reproductive losses can easily be invisible. One couple said they pretended they were not infertile when around friends. Another couple, experiencing a failed in vitro fertilization, felt they lost a child but did not tell anyone else. (We) "didn't want to tell people about it because we were afraid it would fail. It's not like a natural death, when everyone comes forth." In another case, a man said his family did not recognize that their miscarriage meant a child had died. It was just a "mass removed."

Couples may not recognize the loss themselves. One couple said they "played down" the importance of their miscarriage. The husband was not upset by the miscarriage; the wife returned to work immediately. She felt later, though, that she had not dealt with the grief related to the miscarriage because she found herself fantasizing about other children, experiencing anger towards her husband, remembering dates related to the loss, and fearing another pregnancy because it might end in the same manner.

Cultural Factors

Although not identified in the literature as a factor mediating the grief that follows reproductive loss, cultural factors were identified by participants as such. One couple thought that their acceptance of adoption as a method for creating a family was facilitated by the culture surrounding them during their "growing up" years, where creating families through adoption and remarriage were common. They also felt their grief about infertility was therefore not so devastating. Conversely, couples noted that living in a region, such as the South, where strong value is placed on the family is particularly stressful.

Grieving may be worse at specific times identified by a culture as "family times," such as holidays or anniversaries. Christmas was frequently mentioned as a sad time for families experiencing reproductive loss. "Last Christmas was hard. Our child was due in December. All we could think about was we should be planning a birthday party instead of Christmas. Nobody else remembered."

CONCLUSION

Reproductive loss, infertility, miscarriage, and stillbirth, results in the loss of a biological child. Additionally, ten couples interviewed in this study reported five categories of associated losses: the experience of pregnancy, childbirth and breastfeeding; parenting; control; relationships; and one's view of oneself as a fertile individual. Grieving was frequently complicated by the nature of reproductive losses; they usually lack a clear cut time when a loss occurs. The intensity of grieving did change over time, though the impact of the reproductive loss never completely disappeared. Couples experienced the following feelings during the grief process: shock, a sense of unfairness, fear, anger, a sense of being different from others, and intense sadness.

Six factors mediated the grieving process:

1. Multiple losses seemed to increase the intensity and prolong the grief experienced.
2. The quality of existing relationships, between the couple interviewed, other family members, friends, and helping professionals, determined whether the couples felt supported or isolated. Difficult situations were made less so when supportive relationships existed.
3. Whether or not an individual perceived him or herself "responsible" for the loss influenced the amount of support experienced in the relationship. Couples that shared the responsibility and did not blame each other, no matter the reason for the reproductive loss, seemed more resilient.
4. Women and men perceived women to be more impacted by reproductive loss.
5. Couples repeatedly noted that their grieving would be easier if other people recognized the extent of their loss and allowed the couples to talk about their experiences. Commonly, the couples thought they did not recognize the extent of their loss and reported initial attempts to minimize it.
6. Cultural factors, such as specially identified family times and strong values about family, intensified grieving.

This qualitative research project, exploring the experiences of ten couples experiencing reproductive loss, does not allow inferences to others in a similar situation. The sample is select. Each of the couples perceived themselves successful careerwise. It also represents only married couples, and couples that were willing to talk about their experience. Couples who experienced reproductive loss and then separated or those unable or unwilling to participate are not included. The sample does not represent persons who experience reproductive loss for reasons other than the inability to reproduce biologically, such as men and women who wish a biological child but are not in a relationship allowing that. The findings do present the in-depth experiences of ten couples, however, allowing others to learn vicariously about the impact of infertility, miscarriage, and stillbirth.

REFERENCES

Adler, J. (1986, March 24). Learning from the loss. *Newsweek*. 66-67.
Berezin, N. (1982). *After a loss in pregnancy*. New York: Simon and Schuster.
Bierkens, P.B. (1975). Childlessness from the psychological point of view. *Menninger Clinic Bulletin, 39*, 177-182.
Borg, S. & Lasker, J. (1981). *When pregnancy fails*. Boston: Beacon Press.
Bowlby, J. (1980). *Loss: Sadness & depression-attachment & loss. (Vol. III)*. New York: Basic Books.
Brand, H.J. (1982). Die invloed van geslagsver skille op die aanvaarding van infertiliteit. *South African Journal of Psychology, 11*(4), 148-152.
Friedman, R. & Gradstein, B. (1982). *Surviving pregnancy loss*. Boston: Little, Brown and Company.
Hertz, D.G. (1982). Infertility and the physician-patient relationship: A biopsychosocial challenge. *General Hospital Psychiatry, 4*(2), 95-101.
Herz, E. (1984). Psychological repercussions of pregnancy loss. *Psychiatric Annals, 14*(6), 454-457.
Ilse, S. & Burns, L.H. (1985). *Miscarriage: a shattered dream*. Long Lake, MN: Lakeland Press.
Kirkley-Best, E. & Kellner, K.R. (1982). The forgotten grief: A review of the psychology of stillbirth. *American Journal of Orthopsychiatry, 52*(3), 420-427.
Klaus, M.H. & Kennell, J.H. (1976). *Maternal-infant bonding*. Saint Louis: C.V. Mosby Company.
Knapp, R.J. & Peppers, L.G. (1979). Doctor-patient relationships in fetal/infant death encounters. *Journal of Medical Education, 54*, 775-780.
Kraft, A.D., Palombo, J., Mitchell, D., Dean, C. Meyers, S. & Schmidt, A.W. (1980). The psychological dimensions of infertility. *American Journal of Orthopsychiatry, 50*(4), 618-628.
Malloy, M. (1975). *My song for him who never sang to me*. New York: Crown Publishers.
Mazor, M.D. & Simons, H.F. (Eds.). (1984). *Infertility: Medical, emotional and social considerations*. New York: Human Sciences Press, Inc.
Menning, B.E. (1977). *Infertility: A guide for the childless couple*. Englewood Cliffs: Prentice-Hall, Inc.
Menning, B.E. (1980). The emotional needs of infertile couples. *Fertility and Sterility, 34*(4), 313-319.
Palmer, C.E. & Noble, D.N. (1986). Premature death: Dilemmas of infant mortality. *Social Casework: The Journal of Contemporary Social Work, 67*(6), 332-339.
Peppers, L.G. & Knapp, R.J. (1980). *Motherhood and mourning*. New York: Praeger Publishers.
Raphael, B. (1983). *The anatomy of bereavement*. New York: Basic Books, Inc.
Schneider, J. (1984). *Stress, loss and grief*. Baltimore: University Park Press.
Shapiro, C.H. (1982). The impact of infertility on the marital relationship. *Social Casework, 63*(7), 387-393.

Shwartz, D. (1984). When the baby doesn't come home. *Children Today, 13*(2), 21-24.

Silverman, P.R. (1981). *Helping women cope with grief.* Beverly Hills: Sage Publications.

Stringham, J.G., Riley, H. & Ross, A. (1982). Silent birth: Mourning a stillborn baby. *Social Work, 27*(4), 322-327.

Stack, J.M. (1980). Spontaneous abortion and grieving. *American Family Physician, 21*(5), 99-102.

Stack, J.M. (1984). The psychodynamics of spontaneous abortion. *American Journal of Orthopsychiatry, 54*(1), 162-167.

Support to Persons Experiencing Infertility: Family and Friends Can Help

Patricia Payne Mahlstedt
Page Townsend Johnson

SUMMARY. The individual or couple being treated for infertility is emotionally connected to a larger family and social unit which may also feel the sting of infertility. Wanting to help, they often fail because of a lack of understanding of the many losses which accompany infertility, the difficulty in dealing with another's pain, sexual connotations of infertility, and differences in personalities. The authors briefly examine the emotional needs of infertility patients and then identify ways family and friends can provide support.

The emotional assault of infertility — the diagnosis, treatment, and day-to-day experiences — can leave both men and women depressed, angry, and guilt-ridden. These emotional and social consequences impact not only the infertile couple, but also their parents, siblings, friends, coworkers, and even employers. During prolonged diagnoses and treatment, relationships change, and growing numbers of family members and friends agonize over what to say and what to do. Despite their best intentions, they often respond in hurtful ways.

The following scenarios reveal the confusion which infertility creates in relationships:

My best friend has been trying to get pregnant for seven years. She has had surgeries, taken medications, and endured multiple unsuccessful treatments. And now I am pregnant just one year after getting married. I'm afraid to tell her. She may not want to see me.

> My sister can't have children. After I had a baby, she stopped coming by and calling. I don't know what to do.

Frequently family members and friends are unable to provide emotional support because they know so little about the medical and emotional aspects of infertility. With little, often erroneous information, they may not fully comprehend what a devastating loss infertility can be. Comments intended to help can actually sharpen the couple's pain:

> You've got to get hold of yourself.

> You shouldn't feel that way when you have so much to be grateful for.

> Just relax.

> Adopt or quit work and you'll get pregnant. (Statistically, only 5% of all couples who adopt later get pregnant.)

Anecdotal and clinical data confirm that infertility creates multiple hardships in a normal couple's life. The impact of these hardships can be lessened by the responses of a larger family and social network to whom the couple is emotionally connected. Helpful, supportive responses depend on an understanding of the couple's needs and the many losses which accompany infertility.

THE LOSSES OF INFERTILITY

Loss—both real and symbolic—is a major cause of depression. White, Davis, and Cantrell (1977) identify eight types of loss in adulthood, any *one* of which can precipitate depression in the average man or woman: *loss of status, self-esteem, control, important relationships, health or an acceptable body image, security, important fantasies, and someone or something of symbolic value.* Astonishingly, the infertile patient may experience them *all*.

Couples may worry that their status within their peer group is changed as their friends with children develop new interests and activities. This affects the couple's self-esteem, which is further diminished by new, intense, and sometimes very negative feelings;

by the often dehumanizing, embarrassing treatment strategies; by the critical attitudes of others; and by the couple's own nagging belief that they are somehow responsible. Not being able to conceive after trying so hard leads to a sense of being out of control and powerless, unable to achieve what seems so natural and simple. The infertile man or woman struggling with such a damaged self-image and loss of control becomes uncertain that relationships with spouses, family, and friends will survive the pressures of infertility. To compound matters, the couple's sex life becomes less spontaneous and personal, and they may begin to consider themselves "defective." Their perspective on life may even change as they are forced to deal with emotional and financial insecurities and the apparent unfairness of life. Finally, they lose a dream, the fantasy of becoming parents and continuing the cycle of life; to many people, this is the essence of becoming an adult.

The cumulative effect of so many losses is profound, thus creating a major life crisis manifested by feelings of depression, frustration, anger, and guilt. This crisis can become all-consuming with no foreseeable or immediate resolution. It can lead to strained emotional, physical and financial resources, disrupt life goals, intensify past, unresolved problems, and impair relationships. Certainty is lost, control is given to others, and doubt prevails.

The result is that infertile couples become *angry* and *frustrated*, especially in the face of growing child abuse and abortion. They are frustrated by other people's insensitivity, hurt by criticism from their families, tired of medical procedures, upset by limited options and inconclusive diagnoses, and resentful of their fishbowl existence. Stormed one man, "I was furious when I got to the lab to give a sperm sample and was directed to a bathroom with a sign on the door reading 'Sperm Count in Progress.'"

The corker may be that the medical professionals do not agree among themselves about the proper course of treatment and are often insensitive to the couple's need for privacy and concern. After years of trying, one patient finally got pregnant, only to miscarry in her third month. She went to her obstetrician's office later to find out the results of the D&C. He appeared in the doorway of the waiting room and called to her across a room full of pregnant women, "Oh, Mrs. _____, the lab report said it was just a bad egg. Go home and try again." Dealing with infertility on a daily basis, physicians sometimes become desensitized to the highly personal nature of these issues. What is a clinical matter to a physician may be a highly intimate revelation for the couple.

Accompanying the anger is a sense of guilt for being infertile and for being on an emotional roller coaster. Both the man and woman ask themselves: Will the family name end with me? Should I quit work? Did I fail to take care of my body properly? Did I wait too long? Is God punishing me? Am I too upset? Family and friends ask similar questions. The irrational belief that the couple must have caused their infertility exacerbates the couple's sense of blame. Some people respond by pulling away from others, isolating themselves to avoid further pain.

PROVIDING HELP AND SUPPORT

There is no simple remedy to ease such deep pain and extensive loss. Doctors are learning that this emotional suffering can affect a patient's treatment and entire well-being. One Houston endocrinologist suggested, "I think we would see more successful pregnancies if the family and friends of infertile couples knew how to be emotionally supportive." Patients who have support groups, whether it be their family and friends, other infertility patients, or professional help, feel better about themselves and respond better to treatment demands. Those who want to give this support need accurate and specific suggestions for dealing with another person's pain, the sexual connotations of infertility, and the differences in personalities involved.

Become informed. Resolve, Inc., is a national organization which provides information and guidance for infertile couples and their families. Reviewing the Resolve bibliography and asking the couple to share any literature or information they have about their own infertility can be very supportive. This expression of interest often leads to intimate, personal discussion. Support groups of other infertile couples provide help in multiple ways. In addition to those sponsored by Resolve, psychologists and social workers who specialize in infertility offer individual and group counseling. Some people find certain issues too sensitive to discuss with family and friends, and short-term counseling can provide an opportunity for expressing these pent-up frustrations. Physicians who deal with infertility will know about local resources and can make recommendations.

Acknowledge the infertility. Because of the sensitive, highly personal nature of infertility, family and friends feel awkward or embarrassed and so avoid discussing it. Most infertile couples indicate that this is not helpful and only alienates them. Therefore, helpers must come to terms with what infertility means to them, as well as what it means to the couple by examining their own deep-rooted feelings about procreation and medical intervention. For example, potential grandmothers and grandfathers must deal with thwarted expectations of grandchildren and photos on every dresser. Others must ask themselves: Can I really support my child in the choice of treatment and doctor, the decision to adopt, or even the decision to remain child-free? They then must acknowledge the problem to the couple by asking how things are going with treatment, or just by asking how they are feeling. This also demonstrates interest and offers the couple an opportunity to discuss their feelings. If the couple does not elaborate on their activities, further questions are inappropriate at that time. They will at least know what someone recognizes the significance of this experience in their lives.

Be realistic. Often helpers believe that in order to be effective, they must eliminate another's pain. This is unrealistic and often interferes with communication. While caring people cannot take away the couple's pain, they can help them manage it. Those wanting to be helpful must be honest with the couple about their own discomfort and emotional limitations. Potential helpers must share the concern that they may unintentionally say or do hurtful things and then ask the couple for understanding, patience, and guidance. They must ask themselves: Are sexually-related matters open for discussion if the couple decides to confide in me? If I feel overwhelmed, can I tell them? If the couple rejects or ignores my overtures of help, will I be put off or will I reach out to them at another time? Anticipating these situations will enable helpers to handle them with greater confidence. The underlying purpose of any discussion is to communicate concern. It is important to keep that in mind if the discussion gets tense or confuses.

Listen. Helpers must not be afraid of the couple's depression, anger, and guilt. If a couple will talk about their infertility, allow them to freely and fully express their emotions. The couple may deal with these emotions by grieving, a process of crying and repeatedly talking about what has happened and what might happen in the future. By ventilating negative feelings and releasing tension, they can often move on to a more positive, optimistic perspective. Suppressing emotional pain may just delay the grieving process or protract it for those couples who undergo years of treatment. Persons experiencing infertility more often want a sounding board than an opinion.

Recognize different ways of coping. Persons experiencing infertility respond in a variety of ways. They come from divergent economic, religious, and cultural backgrounds, all of which influence their responses to infertility. Some people want to be included in all family and social gatherings which involve children, while others actively avoid such events. Some talk openly about their treatment; others share nothing. Moreover, treatment demands are so varied that the couple's needs change. The woman who is offended because someone asks about her treatment today is the same woman who may be hurt because someone does not ask about it tomorrow. She may talk incessantly about the treatment or condition one time and another time burst into tears at the mention of it. Often a caring friend can only help by doing nothing — a difficult thing to learn.

A husband and wife often have different coping styles and may be in different stages of the grieving process. As a result, it is sometimes difficult to help one of them without alienating the other. As the couple learns to deal with the problem, they will try various methods of coping. Helpers must ask the couple what types of support they need. If they don't know, they should be encouraged to think about what they expect so that they can discuss it. By so doing, the couple recognizes that they are the authority on *what* they need, *when* they need it, and *from whom* they would like to receive it.

Make the invitation. Baby showers, christening, and holidays are especially difficult for the infertile couple. An invitation lets people know they are thought of and wanted. If they choose to decline, accept their choice. It's always nice to be asked.

Accept the couple's need for dignity and respect. Friends and relatives need to let the infertile couple know that they see them as multifaceted people and that infertility is not something that makes them helpless or their lives less meaningful. Helpers must respect the couple's desire for a child, even if they do not agree with the method of attaining that goal. Most importantly, family and friends must reaffirm the couple's importance personally, letting them know that they are loved and accepted, not as an infertile couple, but as a couple who also happens to be infertile.

Infertility is a wound to the body, the mind, and the soul that will not heal properly without the support of someone who cares about the couple and who understands what they are experiencing. Those wanting to help will succeed more often if they are honest about their own values and life goals and open-minded about those of someone else, willing to learn about the multiple losses and stresses of infertility, and prepared to listen. Infertility touches more than the lives of the couple. It can disrupt normal functioning in the family, in the workplace, and in the community. If the current infertility rate continues, the need for knowledgeable and caring support groups will become critical.

REFERENCE

White, R.B., Davis, H.K., & Cantrell, W.A. (1977). Psychodymanics of depression. In G. Usdin (Ed.) *Depression: Clinical, biological and psychological perspectives*. New York: Brunner/Mazel.

Vulnerability to Crises During the Life Cycle of the Adoptive Family

Dorothy W. LePere

SUMMARY. Infertility is a major stressor in the lives of married couples. Recent studies also indicate that adoption understanding is a life crisis for the child adoptee. The losses experienced by adoptive parents and adopted children have an impact not only on the development of these individuals, but also on the family as it meets developmental milestones. Because of the differences in the formation of the adoptive family, the family is more vulnerable to dysfunction over the life cycle than nonadoptive families. This article will explore the nature of these crises and the implications for interventions with the family.

Adoptive family life is complicated, little understood phenomena. It is the position of the author that adoptive families often face crises which are different from those experienced by biologically built families. Adoptive families face these crises alone and with little preparation. In an effort to better understand the factors which lead to successful adoptive parenting, family life crises which are more difficult for the adoptive family are identified and variables related to good adjustment are explored. An examination of normal crises which most families confront throughout the family life cycle are also presented with an analysis of how these are different for the infertile couple, who choose adoption as their option for parenthood.

FAMILY LIFE CYCLE AND MATURATIONAL CRISIS

Just as individuals proceed through a series of predictable, sequential developmental stages, families also experience developmental stages over the family's life cycle. Carter and Mc Goldrick

(1980) identify the following family developmental stages and their corresponding developmental tasks:

Life Cycle Stage	Developmental Tasks
1. The Young Adult	a. Separation from family of origin b. Development of intimate relationships with peers c. Establishment of work identity
2. The Married Couple	a. Establishment of the marital dyad b. Establishment as a couple of successful relationships with others
3. The Family with Young Children	a. Adjustment of the marital relationship to children b. Establishment of parenting roles c. Realignment of relationships with extended family
4. The Family with Adolescents	a. Adjustment of the parent-child relationships to permit the adolescent to develop emotional separation and independence b. Focus on career and marriage c. Realignment of relationship with parents
5. The Empty Nest	a. Realignment of marital relationship b. Establishment of adult relationship with children c. Expansions of relationships to include in-laws and grandchildren

	d. Dealing with disabilities and death of parents
6. The Later Life Family	a. Maintenance of functional relationships and self-functioning while dealing with physical decline
	b. Dealing with significant losses, peers, siblings, spouse, and preparation for own death (p. 17).

These tasks are similar to individual development in that they are related to the development of the independent personality while maintaining closeness and nurturing. Individuals who successfully complete developmental tasks and establish healthy adult personalities are almost always products of families who provide nurturing along with increasing opportunities for independence. The ability of the family to provide nurturing and independence for its members is directly related to the ability of the parents to nurture without stifling the child's desire for separateness and independence from the family. The stages in which healthy families provide increasing independence are those stages in which the individual's development requires increasing responsibility to master the developmental task. Scherz (1971) identified the three primary tasks of the family as (1) emotional separateness vs. interdependences or connectedness; (2) closeness or intimacy vs. other responsibility; and (3) self-autonomy vs. responsibility.

A family's progress through the stages of development is comparable to the individual's progress in that development is complex and does not follow a smooth time line. Families experience a high degree of stress when a new stage of development is eminent. The stress emanates from the conflict between the impetus to progress, the fear of the unknown, and comfortableness of the present stage of development (Scherz, 1971, p. 363). This conflict is often identified as a maturational crisis.

Crises are critical points in the family's development which create an environment which is either conducive to growth or regression depending upon complex factors within the family system.

Shapiro (1982) identifies the expected crises in the family life cycle as those which are related to parent-child interactions. Common crises are the birth of the first child, the first child entering school, adolescence and the last child leaving home.

Scherz (1971) associates the maturational crisis with a mourning process. Mourning takes place as the family members grieve for the loss of the old relationship and behaviors which must be given up if the new task is to be accomplished. Successful mastery depends upon the family's ability to be flexible, stable, and supportive of individual growth. The parents ability to mourn while permitting the child to grow and develop is paramount to the success of the child's development.

THE UNANTICIPATED CRISIS

Infertility is an unanticipated crisis in the family's life. Few are prepared by life experiences or coping mechanisms to respond to the infertility crisis (Shapiro, 1982). Developmental literature on families and individuals does not include a stage for the infertile couple to assimilate and make an adequate adjustment to their loss. In fact, most developmental literature implies that the absence of parenthood or the failure to reproduce, can lead to the lack of full development of the individual personality (Kraft et al., 1980).

Wiehe (1976) maintains that the initial reaction of couples to infertility is so painful that massive denial occurs. His research indicates that it is only after a couple becomes parents that the intensity of their feelings is recognized. Berk and Shapiro (1984) report that infertility and medical tests and procedures are a consuming factor in the couple and individual's life.

Infertile couples frequently express feelings of guilt and unworthiness, lack of self-esteem, diminished sexuality, and associated depression. One study reports that individuals who experienced infertility perceive themselves as less like their ideal selves than matched fertile subjects (Berk & Shapiro, 1984). Many infertile women experience role confusion in that they are unable to fulfill what they perceive to be their primary role, that of motherhood.

Many couples report moderate to severe marital problems related to infertility. While a few couples are able to respond to the infertility crisis in a supportive, empathetic manner, most couples experience significant stress on the marriage, especially in their sexual relationship (Berk & Shapiro 1984). Couples who are actively pursing fertility measures, for example, report a lack of spontaneity in their sexual relationship because of mechanical timing and procedures prescribed by the fertility specialists.

There may also be severe financial strain on the family due to the cost of fertility procedures. The cost of tests and hospitalizations, may be in the thousands of dollars. Couples who pursue pregnancy to the point of in vitro fertilization must pay a minimum of $15,000 for a one-time attempt. In vitro fertilization results in a pregnancy in 7-14% after three attempts. The rates for pregnancies culminating in live births are much lower (Guznick et al., 1986).

The loss or temporary withdrawal of the support to the infertile couple is also stressful. It is difficult to assess whether the isolation is due to withdrawal by the support system or if the depression, anxiety, and emotional turmoil experienced by infertile couples creates a climate in which they avoid and withdraw from friends, family, and others. Mial (1984) reports that infertile subjects perceive negative consequences associated with their disclosure of infertility to others.

Rapoport (1962) emphasizes that crises are experienced as a threat, a loss, or a challenge. Although infertile couples probably experience all three perceptions, the strongest is the sense of loss: loss of biological continuity and of tangible evidence of their existence. Infertile couples must handle their sense of loss through a mourning process. Unfortunately, there are no rituals to observe to mark the end of the couple's hopes of children to be born to this marriage. Shapiro (1982) stresses the need for mourning to achieve a healthy adjustment to infertility.

Often overlooked is the grief of the infertile couple's own parents. They may feel the pain of their child's loss and if there are no other grandchildren, the loss of a biological future for them. They may feel helpless in the face of their children's pain and retreat from the couple just at the time the couple needs them most (Shapiro, 1982). The infertile couple may interpret this retreat as another rejection and experience added grief from the estrangement from their families of origin.

If the infertile couple can successfully mourn their loss, they may be able to consider alternatives for parenthood or a child-free life style. Shapiro (1982) suggests that acceptance may be reached at different times for each individual in the marital partnership. She stresses that acceptance of one's infertility does not mean that the pain of infertility is gone, but it does decrease and preoccupation with childlessness is no longer so intense.

Kraft, et al. (1980) identifies three tasks that infertile couples must accomplish as they adapt to infertility:

1. Acknowledge the injury of missing a basic life experience;
2. Restore a healthy body image; and
3. Assess the importance of parenthood and determine if other activities compensate, consider other forms of parenthood (p. 623).

The self-concepts of the persons who experience infertility are thus reorganized around issues other than fertility if the couple is to make a good adjustment. If this adaptation is not made, the couple is not only less successful handling the crisis, but is also less likely to successfully master subsequent developmental stages and tasks of the family life cycle. This clearly has implications for adoptive parenthood. Couples who do not make this adjustment are not considered good candidates for adoptive parenting (Kraft, et al., 1980).

THE ADOPTIVE COUPLE:
PROGRESS THROUGH THE LIFE CYCLE

It appears that the ability to parent is not affected for those couples who make an adequate adjustment to infertility and choose adoption. While there may be unique family stressors experienced by the adoptive family that the family with birth children does not experience, research suggests that adoptive parents are as accepting and as competent as other families. Anderson (1978), found that adoptive fathers are not as likely as birth fathers to feel that it is impossible to change a child's behavior. Adoptive fathers were more likely to believe that parental influences are as important as hereditary factors. She also found that adoptive parents are more accepting of children's behaviors and feelings and more trusting of their children than biological parents. Kraft, et al. (1980) believe that the infertile couples who are most successful are those who had stable childhoods and strong, caring parents who were empathetic to their needs. This would explain their ability to be accepting and trusting of their adopted children.

Ternay and Wilborn (1985) report that adoptive families are no different from families who give birth to children when the parents are compared on the basis of general personal adjustment and parental behaviors. Gease (1982) found that adoptive families of children who had problems were less conflicted than biological families with similar types of children.

If adoptive parents have adjusted to their infertility, if they have good parenting abilities and are as well-adjusted as the general population, what contributes to the adoptive family's vulnerability to crisis? The key issues appear to be "loss" and differences in how the family was built.

Despite the joyous outcome, infertile, adoptive parents must look forward to a more stressful parenting experience than the fertile couple. Both the individual and the family are at risk for crisis at points in the life cycle. The most critical points for the adoptive family appear to be:

1. The period while the adoption study is being conducted. This includes the rigor of making application, attending preparation classes and participating in the home study process;
2. The waiting period after successful completion of the adoption study and placement of the child;
3. The time of actual placement of the adopted child;
4. The waiting period after the child is placed prior to legalization;
5. The adoption revelation process;
6. When the adopted child enters school;
7. When the adopted child understands the abstract loss which he or she has experienced;

8. When the adopted child, at adolescence, begins to question his or her biological origins; and
9. When the adopted adult marries and bears children.

The adoption study process typically engenders anxiety of prospective adoptive parents. Pendarvis (1985) found that the couple's anxiety is actually higher while waiting for the study to be performed than during or after the home study is conducted. These feelings are similar to the feelings experienced during the infertility testing period. The study itself is also stressful, however. Feelings of insecurity are aroused as the family is subjected to outside scrutiny and interventions not required of biological parents. On an emotional level the adoption study process is similar to fertility procedures the couple has experienced. Adoptive parents must "pay their dues" and be "approved" to be parents (Berman & Bufferd, 1986).

Adoptive parents may also experience a postpartum reaction after the child is placed. Berman and Bufferd (1986) maintain that this postpartum depression can be attributed to the fact that adoptive parents must once again confront their infertility. The adopted child is tangible proof that the couple could not give birth to a child. The couple faces the loss of biological parenthood and grieve for this loss. The adoptive family must acknowledge that adoption is a cure for childlessness but not for infertility.

In almost every case, a couple must wait a minimum of six months before legal adoption of the child can take place. During this time, most jurisdictions require supervision by the agency or the court to determine whether the adoptive parents are adequate. This period may interfere with the family's feeling of entitlement and responsibility for the adopted child (Berman & Bufferd, 1986).

Adoption authorities advise the adoptive parents to tell the child that he or she is adopted at three or four-years-old. Brodzinsky, Schechter, Braff and Singer (1984) maintain that this is a particularly stressful time for adoptive parents. They criticize the information and training provided to adoptive parents in this area on the basis of its inadequacy. It only provides a very elementary outline of the information necessary to support adoptive parents during the adoption and revelation process. They believe that adoptive parents find this experience so stressful, that the child may only be told briefly about his or her adoption as a preschooler. When the child is older and asks more in-depth, detailed questions, the parents are ill-prepared or uncomfortable.

Many families report that the time when their first child enters school is very stressful. Adoptive parents may find that as their adopted child begins school, feelings of loss are relived. Because of their loss through infertility, other losses and separations are more painful. An additionally powerful reminder of infertility and adoption status pertains to the fact that enrollment in school may be the first time parents have had to use the child's birth certificate. This certificate may even be identified as a birth certificate issued through adoption.

Brodzinsky, Schechter, Braff and Singer (1984) identify latency as the time in which the adopted child begins to understand that to be adopted, one must have first lost a set of parents. Adoptive parents may not be prepared for this grief. They may feel that the "adoption issue" was "handled" when the child was a pre-schooler. Berman and Bufferd (1986) believe that adopted children have no means to adequately mourn the loss of their birth parents and support by the adoptive parents may not be available. The knowledge that their child is grieving for another set of parents is very painful for the adoptive parents. The existential grief experienced by adopted children may account for the problems seen in school-aged adopted children. Brodzinsky et al. (1984) reports that adopted children are more prone to psychological and school-related behavior problems. Berman and Bufferd (1986) relate these problems to the school-aged child's anger, depression, and guilt associated with the loss of the birth parents. The child may also harbor fear of another rejection by the adoptive parents.

Adolescence has always been identified as the most difficult time for the adopted family. Sorosky et al. (1975) identify early adolescence as the time the adopted child is able to conceptualize the biological link between generations. Adolescence is a stressful time for all families, compounded in adoptive families by the need of the adopted child to develop some biological continuity. Adoptive parents may be threatened by this curiosity. They may fear that seeking information about the birth parents is a rejection of them as parents.

Colon (1978) maintains that the adolescent adoptee's need to know is often unrelated to the strength of the relationship with the adoptive parents. One recent study, however has indicated that adults who seek contact with birth parents are less likely to have identified with the adoptive mother (Lamski, 1980). Adoptive parents may also be uncomfortable with the adolescent's awakening sexuality. The adoptive parents may fear an unplanned, unwanted pregnancy especially if their child's birth parents were unmarried. The fertility of their child also once again brings the couple face-to-face with their own infertility.

The adolescent's struggle for independence is seen by most parents as a loss. For the adoptive parents, this loss is more complex and their adolescent's strivings for independence may be especially difficult to handle. With independence comes separation. Adoptive parents may attempt to keep their child too close and not allow the adolescent to adequately separate and develop autonomy. The adopted adolescent may also have difficulty separating from his or her parents from fear of rejection or abandonment by the adopted family.

The last period of increased vulnerability during the family life cycle for the adoptive family is the marriage and birth of grandchildren. Not only is the couple again reminded of their infertility, they must also recognize that attachment to their grandchildren is not based on hereditary factors.

THE SUCCESSFUL FAMILY

If adoption itself coupled with infertility make the adopted child and his or her family more vulnerable to crises, how do adoptive families handle these unique stressors? A number of studies report that these vulnerabilities translate to an adopted child's having an increased likelihood of school and behavior problems than the general population. Brodzinsky et al. (1984) view these problems as developmentally-specific issues that do not carry over to the adoptee's later life. Kirk et al. (1966) maintain, however, that most studies relating to adopted children are not matched closely enough to afford valid information about the long-term effects of adoption on the child and his or her family.

It is likely however, that adoptive families do have more difficulty negotiating and mastering the developmental tasks through the life cycle. Suggestions have been proposed to explain successful adoptive parenting. Kraft et al. (1980) relate successful adoption to a good adjustment to the infertility crisis. Kirk (1981) believes that families who are able to see adoptive parenthood as different from biological parenthood are more successful than those who reject differences. The Brodzinsky et al. (1984) research indicates that families who handle adoption revelation on a continuing basis are more successful. Sorosky et al. (1975) associate successful adoption with acceptance of the birth parents and information sharing by the adoptive parents including assisting in the search.

Family life cycle theorists assert that families who master one developmental task successfully are more likely to handle the next maturational milestone successfully. Thus, the adjustment the couple makes to their infertility would be linked to subsequent successful parenting. Family theorists strongly emphasize that open family communications are essential for the family's progress from one stage of development to another (Scherz, 1971). This addresses issues pertaining to adoption revelation and open discussion of the child's biological origins.

In essence, adoptive parenting strains the emotional resources of the couple. In order for the family to meet the developmental crisis with growth rather than regression, the adoptive parents need the ability to grieve their losses. They need to be strong, stable individuals who are flexible enough to learn from their own experiences and the experiences of other adoptive parents.

RECOMMENDATIONS

The author focuses on the infertile couple who choose adoption as an alternative to childlessness. It is hypothesized that fertile couples who choose to adopt a child will face some of the same stressors without the burden of infertility. Also, families who choose to adopt older children will necessarily have similar and additional stressors related to missing some of the child's and family's developmental milestones. Both situations could provide additional data about the role of adoption in the family life cycle.

In addition to examining the adoptive parents' abilities to make an adequate adjustment to infertility and adoption, the adoption system and the general support provided to adoptive families must be examined. While public attitudes are most difficult to change, the ways in which families become adoptive parents should be closely examined. Four basic changes in the system are recommended:

1. The study process must help the family recognize their grief about their infertility and make an adequate adjustment to this grief;
2. The study process should be designed such that the family's anxiety is lessened as much as possible;
3. Education about the differences in adoptive family life must be an essential part of the preparation process. Information about the continuum of adoption revelation should be discussed with the adoptive family so that the family is not surprised or hurt by the child's behavior in latency and adolescence; and
4. Ongoing support for adoptive families at critical points in the family life cycle is essential in promoting mastery of difficult developmental milestones.

In summary, adoptive families are more vulnerable to problems in the family life cycle because of the nature of the way the family was built. Research indicates that these problems are not insurmountable, but that adoptive families can benefit from support, careful attention and preparation. As in any family, the adoptive families who are most likely to be successful are those who learn to resolve problems through open communication, who are able to provide nurturing while fostering independence, and who have a secure sense of themselves as capable members of families.

REFERENCES

Anderson, J. (1978). Child rearing attitudes, perceived parental behavior patterns and learning disabilities in adoptive and natural families. Unpublished doctoral dissertation, North Texas State University, Denton.

Berk, A. & Shapiro, J.L. (1984). Some implications of infertility on marital therapy. *Family Therapy, 11*.

Berman, L.C. & Bufferd, R.K. (1986). Family treatment to address loss in adoptive families. *Social Casework, 67*, 3-11.

Brodzinsky, D.M., Schechter, D.E., Braff, A.M. & Singer, L.M. (1984). Psychological and academic adjustment in adopted children. *Journal of Consulting and Clinical Psychology*, *52*, 582-590.

Carter, E. & McGoldrich, M. (1980). *The family life cycle: A framework for family therapy*. New York: Gardner.

Colon, F. (1978). Family ties and child placement. *Family Process*, *17*, 289-312.

Gease, E.I. (1982). *Adoptive families evaluated by a court diagnostic team*. Unpublished doctoral dissertation, University of Maryland, Baltimore.

Guznick, D., Wilkes, C. & Jones, H. (1986). Cumulative pregnancy rates for in vitro fertilization. *Fertility and Sterility, 46*, October.

Kirk, H.D. (1981). *Adaptive Kinship: A Modern Institution in Need of Reform*. Toronto: Butterworth Co.

Kirk, H.D., Johassohn, K. & Fish, A., (1966). Are adopted children especially vulnerable to stress? *Archives of General Psychiatry, 14*, 291-298.

Kraft, A., Palombo, J., Mitchell, D., Dean, C., Meyers, S. & Schmidt, A. (1980). The psychological dimensions of infertility. *American Journal of Orthopsychiatry, 50*, 618-628.

Lamski, D.J. (1980). *The search for identity: A problem of the adopted child*. Unpublished doctoral dissertation, California School of Professional Psychology, San Francisco.

Mial, C.E. (1984). Women and involuntary childlessness: Perceptions associated with infertility. Unpublished doctoral dissertation. York University, North York Ontario, Canada.

Pendarvis, L.V. (1985). *Anxiety levels of involuntarily infertile couples*. Unpublished doctoral dissertation, The Ohio State University, Columbus.

Rapoport, L. (1962). The state of crisis: Some theoretical considerations. *Social Service Review, 36*, June.

Scherz, F. (1971). Maturational crises and parent-child interaction. *Social Casework, 63*.

Shapiro, C.H. (1982). The impact of infertility on the marital relationship. *Social Casework, 63*, 387-393.

Sorosky, A., Baran, A. & Pannor, R. (1975). Identity conflicts in adoptees. *American Journal of Orthopsychiatry, 45*, 18-27.

Ternay, M. & Wilborn, B. (1985). Perceived child-parent relationships and child adjustment in families with both adopted and natural children. *Journal of Genetic Psychology, 146*, 261-272.

Wiehe, V. (1976). Psychological reaction to infertility. *Psychological Reports,, 38*, 863-866.

The Institution of Adoption:
Its Sources and Perpetuation

Leroy H. Pelton

SUMMARY. Historical adoption trends are examined in the context of changing child welfare policies (including the permanency planning movement), the social circumstances and causes of the surrender of children for adoption, and women's rights. The focus is on the "front end" of the adoption system, including the perspectives of the birth parents and the range of options that were available to them at the time of surrender. The nature of the relationship between poverty and adoption is explored.

The separation of children from their parents has taken many forms, but none has been more extreme than the modern version of adoption. In adoption, the state has sanctioned the complete severance of all parental rights and responsibilities, as well as of all contact between the parents and child, and the withholding of all knowledge about each other from both the parents and child. While adoption, in this extreme form, might have been practiced at other times and in other places, it is really a very recent phenomenon in the Western world, having been practiced as such, with some gradual loosening of secrecy requirements, for only the past 50 years.

By contrast, in foster care, the prospect exists that the child and parents will be reunited after the factors that have seemingly necessitated the separation have been ameliorated. And in theory, if not always in practice, the child and parents have the right to know the physical location of each other, and can visit and be in written and telephone contact with each other. Moreover, the parents must be consulted in regard to medical decisions concerning the child. Other forms of separation of children from living parents, of course, such as giving them to relatives to raise, hospitalization, or sending them to boarding school or summer camp, do not involve relinquishment of legal rights or responsibilities, do permit continued contact and communication between children and parents and are usually temporary arrangements.

From this perspective, adoption is a peculiar institution. It is quite different from more limited forms of separation that ostensibly serve the most basic and obvious reason for separation at all – to allow the child to be cared for when the parents presumably cannot or will not do so, or to enhance the development of the child.

The institution of adoption would not exist, obviously, if there were not a source of children for it, as well as willing receivers for this ultimate form of child transference. The purpose of this discussion is to explore the changing nature of the source, and the possible factors and reasons involved in the relinquishment of children (by mothers) for adoption.

Relatively speaking, not much has been written, and not much research done, on this "front end" of the adoption system. Indeed, as other commentators have noted, a remarkable feature of the literature on adoption is the extent to which it has avoided discussion of the reasons why parents relinquish children for adoption. By far, the greater proportion of the literature has concerned the development of the adoptive child, the adjustment within the adoptive family, how-to advice for potential adoptive parents, and most recently, the sealed vs. open records controversy. But here it is asked: Where do the children come from, and why are they relinquished?

THE SHIFTING SOURCES OF CHILDREN FOR ADOPTION

Our concern here is with adoptions by nonrelatives. The other type, related adoptions, most often involves the adoption of a child by his or her stepfather, in which separation from the mother does not occur. The majority of adoptions are related, but since they usually do not have the characteristics mentioned above, we will focus on nonrelated adoptions, as does most adoption research.

The annual number of nonrelated adoptions in the United States rose rather steadily from an estimated 33,800 in 1951 to a peak of 89,200 in 1970, and then, more abruptly, declined to an estimated

47,700 in 1975, the last year for which statistics were collected by the National Center for Social Statistics. These estimates, as summarized recently by Maza (1984), are presented in Table 1. The best more recently available estimate, derived from a national survey conducted by the National Committee for Adoption for the year 1982, indicates that the annual number of adoptions might have reached another turning point, rising slightly since 1975 to 50,720 (National Committee for Adoption, 1985; see Table 1). There is independent corroboration from another source of data that there has been a slight increase since 1975 (Bachrach, 1986). From these statistics, it is apparent that there are currently well over two million living Americans who have been adopted by nonrelated parents.

Most commentators agree that the major factors responsible for the overall decline in nonrelated adoptions since 1970 include the decreased social stigmatization of unwed mothers in our society, the increased availability of contraceptives, and the legalization of

Table 1. Estimates of Total Nonrelated Adoptions and Public Agency Adoptions in the United States, and Public Agency Adoptions as a Percentage of Total Nonrelated Adoptions, for 1951-1982.

Year	Total Nonrelated Adoptions	Public Agency Adoptions	Public Agency Percentage
1951	33,800	6,100	18%
1955	48,400	9,700	20
1957	48,200	10,600	22
1958	50,900	10,200	20
1959	54,100	11,400	21
1960	57,800	13,300	23
1961	61,600	15,400	25
1962	62,900	14,500	23
1963	67,300	17,500	26
1964	71,600	18,600	26
1965	76,700	20,700	27
1966	80,600	23,400	29
1967	83,700	23,100	30
1968	86,300	26,800	31
1969	88,900	28,400	32
1970	89,200	29,500	33
1971	82,800	29,800	36
1972	67,300	25,600	38
1973	59,200	22,500	38
1974	49,700	19,400	39
1975	47,700	18,600	39
1982	50,720	19,428	38

Sources: Maza (1984) for 1951-1975, and National Committee for Adoption (1985) for 1982.

abortion (the U.S. Supreme Court struck down anti-abortion laws in 1973). This decline took place despite the fact that the annual number of illegitimate births had risen dramatically, more than doubling between 1957 and 1974 (Bonham, 1977).

National statistics for the United States are also available, for the same years noted above, in regard to the routes through which nonrelated adoptions have been accomplished. In Table 1, we see a rough parallel between the trend for total nonrelated adoptions and that number effected through public agencies: that is, there is a gradual annual increase up until 1970-1971, and then a decline through 1975. There is a slight increase between 1975 and 1982 (Maza, 1984; National Committee for Adoption, 1985). Another survey, by the American Public Welfare Association (APWA) (Tatara & Pettiford, 1985) estimates between 22,000 and 24,000 adoptions nationwide in fiscal year 1982, but is based on data from only 29 states. The National Committee estimate of 19,428 is used here, however, because it is based on direct, unadjusted statewide reports from 32 states. The APWA survey estimates between 19,000 and 21,000 adoptions in fiscal year 1983, based on data from 42 states. As a proportion of all nonrelated adoptions, public agency adoptions rose rather continuously from 18% in 1951 to 39% in 1975, with only a possible minor decline to 38% in 1982 (see Table 1).

The remaining proportion of nonrelated adoptions were effected through the routes of private agency and independent adoptions. Not shown here, but available from Maza's (1984) summary of estimates, is the fact that while independent adoptions predominated proportionately over private agency adoptions from 1951 through 1961, private agency adoptions predominated from 1962 to 1975, hitting its peak of 45% in 1970. Yet the National Committee for Adoption estimates indicate another reversal since 1975 (National Committee for Adoption, 1985, Table 8). In 1975, 39% of nonrelated adoptions were through public agencies, 38% through private agencies, and 23% were independent. In 1982, the percentages were 38% public, 29% private, and 33% independent. It is clear that while there have been fluctuations in the division of nonpublic agency adoptions between private agency and independent, the public agency's proportion has remained at its highest of 38% — 39% since 1972, and has constituted the highest proportion of all three routes since 1974.

It would seem that unlike public agencies, the fortunes of private agencies, in regard to adoptions, rose and fell with their ability to deliver healthy white infants to prospective adoptive parents. Prospective parents for such infants then turned to independent means, and the private agencies were left with a decreasing proportion of a decreasing pie. The public agencies, although not having reached the numbers of adoptions they effected during 1970-1971, have held their own in terms of the proportion of the total pie due to another factor, the permanency planning movement, the effects of which will be discussed shortly. First, one other set of statistics that is available on a trend basis, that for adoptions of foreign children into the United States, will be discussed.

Foreign Adoptions

Adoptions of children from foreign countries began as a trickle in the post-World War II years. From 314 in 1949 and 189 in 1950, the number reached almost 3,000 in 1959 (Krichefsky, 1961). It averaged less than 2,000 per year through the 1960s, and then climbed until the mid-1970s. The figures for federal fiscal year (FY) 1976 through FY 1985 are shown in Table 2 (Immigration and Naturalization Service, 1980, Table 12[1]). For the last five years, the number has risen steadily, to 9,286 in 1985, the highest number of annual foreign adoptions in our country's history, representing a 91% increase since 1981. In 1982, foreign adoptions represented 11.3% of all nonrelated adoptions. If the total number of nonrelated adoptions remained steady since 1982, save for the rise in foreign adoptions, then foreign adoptions would have constituted as much as 17% of all nonrelated adoptions in 1985.

In the post-World War II years, almost all foreign adoptions came from European war-torn countries, mostly from Greece, Germany, and Italy (Krichefsky, 1961). Beginning in 1953, Japan and South Korea became significant contributors to this stream of foreign adoptions (Krichefsky, 1961; Adams & Kim, 1971). By about 1958, South Korea had become the largest single contributor to foreign adoptions in the United States (Krichefsky, 1961), and has remained so up until the present time (Weil, 1984; Immigration and Naturalization Service, 1980, Table 12[1]). By 1976, 59% of all foreign adoptions were coming from South Korea and only 3% from

Table 2. Estimates of Total Foreign Adoptions in The United States, and from the Ten Leading Source Countries in FY 1985, for FY 1976-FY 1985. Figures in Parentheses Represent Percentages of Total Foreign Adoptions.

	FY1976	FY1977	FY1978	FY1979	FY1980	FY1981	FY1982	FY1983	FY1984	FY1985
South Korea	3,859	3,858	3,045	2,406	2,683	2,444	3,254	4,412	5,157	5,694 (61.3)
Colombia	554	575	599	626	653	628	534	608	595	622 (6.7)
Phillipines	323	325	287	297	253	278	345	302	408	515 (5.5)
India	22	85	149	231	319	314	409	409	468	496 (5.3)
El Salvador	86	132	98	139	179	224	199	240	364	310 (3.3)
Brazil	25	39	15	25	48	62	72	55	117	242 (2.6)
Chile	17	24	36	90	92	106	113	172	153	206 (2.2)
Honduras	36	29	24	19	20	13	22	97	148	181 (1.9)
Guatemala	42	52	51	75	75	82	98	105	110	175 (1.9)
Mexico	127	156	152	139	144	116	98	110	168	137 (1.5)
Total: Ten Countries--	5,091 (77.7)	5,275 (81.2)	4,456 (83.8)	4,047 (83.2)	4,466 (86.9)	4,267 (87.7)	5,144 (89.5)	6,510 (91.3)	7,688 (92.3)	8,578 (92.4)
Total: All Countries--	6,552	6,493	5,315	4,864	5,139	4,868	5,749	7,127	8,327	9,286

Sources: Immigration And Naturalization Service, 1980, Table 12; Note 1.

Europe. Colombia was the second highest contributor with 8.5% of the total, and Vietnam was third highest with 6.5% of the total (Immigration and Naturalization Service, 1980, Table 12).

In 1985, a total of ten countries accounted for 92% of all foreign adoptions (see Table 2). In that year, South Korea provided more foreign adoptions than any previous year and by itself accounted for 61% of all foreign adoptions.[1] Colombia, while providing only 6.7% of the total, has contributed more than 500 adoptions per year since 1976. The Philippines surpassed 500 adoptions for the first time. India, which provided only 22 children in 1976, increased rapidly to its high of 496 in 1985. El Salvador supplied more than three and a half times as many children in 1985 as it did in 1976. Brazil increased from only 15 children in 1976 to 119 in 1984 and then more than doubled its contribution in one year's time. Chile's contribution rose from only 17 children in 1976 to over 200 in 1985. Honduras contributed only 22 children as late as 1982, but 181 by 1985. Guatemala surpassed 100 only by 1983 and reached its high point of 175 in 1985. Finally, Mexico has remained around 100 since 1976.

The trends are clear. A handful of developing countries, in Asia and Latin America, are providing almost all of the foreign adoptions to the United States. In 1980, Europe was a source of less than 1% of such adoptions.

In European and other developed countries, too, the influx of foreign adoptions has been mounting, and their sources are also Asia and Latin America. In 1980, for example, 96% of Sweden's 1,703 foreign adoptions for that year came from Asia and Latin America (Pilotti, 1985). France and Germany have adopted from Latin America (Goldschmidt, 1986), and Australia has received children primarily from Asian countries (Fopp, 1982).

In the Netherlands, domestic adoptions outnumbered foreign adoptions by better than five to one in 1967 when there were only 129 foreign adoptions. By 1973, there was roughly an equivalent number of foreign and domestic adoptions, and by 1980, foreign adoptions totaled almost 1,600, and outnumbered domestic adoptions by better than 15 to one (Hoksbergen, 1981). Most came from South Korea, Colombia, India, Indonesia, and Bangladesh.

Although the United States has been the largest receiver of foreign children for adoption in terms of numbers (Weil, 1984), other countries, such as the Netherlands, have been larger receivers in proportion to their population size: Thus Sweden, which had only about 100 domestic children available for adoption each year during the 1970s received from 1,500 to 2,000 foreign children for adoption in each of those years, a third or more of the number that was going to the United States at that time, even though Sweden had only 4% of the population size of the United States (Weil, 1984).

Permanency Planning

From the late 1950s, many studies and reports began to call attention to serious faults in the foster care system in the United States (see, e.g., Maas & Engler, 1959; Maas, 1969; Wald, 1976; Fanshel & Shinn, 1978; Shyne & Shroeder, 1978; Gruber, 1978). At the same time, the number of children in foster care in this country began to grow enormously, reaching its high point of an estimated 500,000 children during 1975-1977 (Knitzer et al., 1978; Shyne & Shroeder, 1978; Pelton, 1987).

Due to eventual alarm over the large number of children in foster care, and mounting professional criticism that they stay too long and move too much, "permanency planning" became a broad and popular movement within the child welfare field during the mid to late 1970s, and later became a major aspect of the federal Adoption Assistance and Child Welfare Act (AACWA) of 1980 (P.L. 96-272). Basically, it was the belief that many children were being harmed by a system in which they stayed indefinitely and drifted from one home to another, without close monitoring of their cases and without plans for more permanent and stable living arrangements, that led to the establishment of permanency planning programs in child welfare agencies, and mechanisms for periodic review of children in foster care guided by a permanency planning philosophy.

The main thrust of the permanency planning movement has been aimed at children already in foster care: to either get them returned home or, if this is deemed not possible, freed for adoption. While some commentators wish to expand the concept of permanency planning to include the prevention of foster care placement in the first instance (Stein & Gambrill, 1985), the reality is that the Oregon Permanency Planning Demonstration Project, which has served as a model for the movement, dealt with children already in foster care, and the emphasis was on adoption (Emlen et al., 1978). Moreover, permanency planning units in public child welfare agencies usually deal with children already in foster care, and most external review mechanisms developed in the last decade are also so focused, and indeed are often called foster care review boards.

In fact, as far back as 1969 (in New York State) but mainly during the 1970s, states passed laws to provide adoption subsidies in order to facilitate the adoption of so-called "hard-to-place" children out of foster care. The AACWA of 1980 introduced federal money into adoption subsidies, in order to facilitate permanency planning efforts. Also, within the past decade, many states have "liberalized" their laws concerning termination of parental rights in order to make it easier to free children for adoption.

While it is true that the AACWA of 1980 states that "reasonable efforts will be made prior to the placement of a child in foster care, to prevent or eliminate the need for removal of the child from his home" and provides federal fiscal incentives for prevention-of-placement services, the proliferation of class action suits in the last few years to attempt to force state and local governments to make such "reasonable efforts" indicates that such efforts have been lacking[2] (Pelton). Indeed, there are indications that the decline in the foster care population that did take place between 1977 and 1982 may be attributable more to an increase in the number of children who exited from foster care than to a decrease in the number who entered, and that the rise in the foster care population in 1983 is due to a continuing failure to deal with the "front end" of the foster care system (Pelton, 1987).

What impact has the advent of the permanency planning philosophy had on adoption trends? As previously noted, the annual number of adoptions through public agencies rose until its high point in 1970-1971 and declined until 1975, with a slight increase shown in 1982 over 1975. Thus, although national estimates are not available for the years 1976-1981, the estimates that are available indicate that the permanency planning movement, at the very least, halted the decline in public agency adoptions during those years.

The permanency planning movement also played a role in the dramatic change that has occurred in the characteristics and indeed the sources of children placed for adoption through the public agencies. In 1971, the median age of children involved in public agency adoptions in the United States (based on data from 36 states) was only four months (that is, 50% of the children adopted were under four months); 73% of the children were under one year, and only 7% were six-years old or more (National Center for Social Statistics, 1973). In FY 1983 (based on data from 24 states), the median age of children whose adoptions were finalized through public agencies was 5.6 years; only 12.7% were under one year, and 46.8% were six-years old or more (Tatara & Pettiford, 1985).

Most of the children headed for adoption in 1971 obviously could not have spent much time in foster care, since they were adopted as infants. Now, most of the children being adopted through public agencies have been residing in the foster care system for several years. Indeed, in New Jersey, for example, 68% of adoptive home placements in 1985 were with foster parents, as compared with only 27% in 1970.[3]

Other characteristics of the children have also changed. In New Jersey, for example, 31% of the public agency adoptive placements in 1970 were of nonwhite children, compared to 68% in 1985.[3] In Tennessee, the nonwhite percentage was 10% in state fiscal year (SFY) 1970 compared to 25% in SFY 1985.[4] As we shall see later, an increasing proportion of adoptive placements involve handicapped children, but the statistics showing this are available for only the last few years.

Three distinct stages in this overall transformation are discernible. The first occurred between 1971 and 1974, at a time when total nonrelated adoptions as well as the number of public agency adoptions were declining, and during a time when the foster care population was increasing considerably. An age increase in public agency adoptions took place that in some states, at least, was due not only to a decline in the availability of white infants for adoption, but also to an apparent informal permanency planning movement that focused on efforts to get older foster children adopted. The median age of children in New Jersey whose adoptions were finalized through the public agency was a mere 5.6 months in 1971 (National Center for Social Statistics, 1973). By 1973, it had jumped to 15.4 months, and as early as SFY 1974, children six years of age and older constituted 47% of all New Jersey public agency adoptive placements (National Center for Social Statistics, 1975[3]).

This change could not have been due to the decline in availability of white infants alone. Nationwide, only 7% of public agency adoptions in 1971 were of children six years of age and older (National Center for Social Statistics, 1973). If we apply this statistic to New Jersey, we can estimate that only 48 children in that age group were placed for adoption through the public agency in 1971.[3] In SFY 1974, however, 188 children in that age group were placed for adoption in New Jersey.[3] Thus an increased number, as well as proportion, of the children were in that age group, indicating that special efforts were being made.

In Tennessee, however, a far more modest change occurred during this period, while its total adoptive placements plummeted. The median age of children involved in adoptive placements rose from 4.0 months in 1971 to 4.4 months in 1974 (National Center for Social Statistics, 1973, 1976). Its adoptive placements of children six years of age and older went from 5% or 28 children, in SFY 1970, to 17%, or 48 children in SFY 1974.[4]

Nevertheless, the evidence suggests that the permanency planning philosophy began to imbue the child welfare field before the mid-1970s. The permanency planning movement began as a thrust to get children adopted, and it did so, at least in some states, as soon as a downturn started in the number of white infants available for adoption.

The next two stages involve the formal permanency planning movement, the first during the mid to late 1970s, and the second after the passage of the AACWA in 1980. In New Jersey, children six years of age and older constituted 47% of public agency adoptive placements in SFY 1974, 57% in SFY 1977, 46% in 1980, and 56% in 1985.[3] In Tennessee, children in this age category constituted 17% of such placements in SFY 1974, 30% in SFY 1977, 19% in SFY 1978, 31% in SFY 1980, and 51% in SFY 1984. Thus we see the impact of the permanency planning movement's push to get older children adopted, a slackening off of that impact after 1977, but then a bolstering of permanency planning efforts by the AACWA, after 1980.

The New Jersey statistics indicate that the proportion of children placed in adoptive homes who were nonwhite was 42% in SFY 1974, 50% in SFY 1977, 51% in 1980, and 68% in 1985.[3] The APWA statistics, based on 30 states, indicate a substantial rise from FY 1982 to FY 1983 (from 30% to 43%) in the proportion of public agency finalized adoptions involving nonwhite children (Tatara & Pettiford, 1985). Thus again the impact of the permanency planning movement and then of AACWA is evident.

Finally, in New Jersey, the proportion of public agency adoptive placements involving children with handicapping conditions (children with a physical handicap, mental retardation, severe emotional disturbances, and multiple handicaps) was 32% in 1982, and 37% in 1985.[3] The APWA data based on 24 states indicate that the proportion of public agency finalized adoptions involving children with "special needs" (including age, disability, and minority or sibling group status) rose from 38% in FY 1982 to 61% in FY 1983 (Tatara & Pettiford, 1985).

We may conclude that the permanency planning movement halted the decline of public agency adoptions, by way of increased efforts to get older and nonwhite children adopted out of the foster care system, but lost some steam in the late 1970s. The faltering movement was then given a shot in the arm by the AACWA of 1980 (which itself was a result of the permanency planning movement). The AACWA was then responsible for a sharp rise in the percentage of children placed for adoption who are older, minority, and handicapped. In New Jersey, more than two-thirds of the children placed for adoption in 1985 were nonwhite, over one half were age six or more, and more than one third were handicapped. The characteristics of children placed for adoption through public agencies have changed drastically.

A major mechanism by which such change was effected was the state adoption subsidy, and then federal participation in subsidies after 1980. The boost that was given to the permanency planning movement by the AACWA was primarily accomplished through that Act's provision of federal money for adoption subsidies. In Illinois, for example, subsidized adoptions as a proportion of all public agency adoptions rose from 41% in SFY 1978 to 48% in SFY 1980, and then to 70% in SFY 1985 (Testa & Lawlor, 1985, p. 55). In Tennessee, subsidized adoptive placements as a proportion of all public agency adoptive placements rose from only 11% in SFY 1977 to 26% in SFY 1980, and to 42% by SFY 1985.[4] In New Jersey, this proportion climbed from 48% in 1977 to 61% in 1979, dropped to 52% in 1980, and then jumped to 83% in both 1984 and 1985.[3] Subsidies are often used to transform the same foster home in which a child had been residing into an adoptive home. In Tennessee, the proportion of adoptive placements that were with foster parents rose from 32% in SFY 1982 to 42% in SFY 1985, the same proportion of placements given adoption subsidies in that year.[4] In New Jersey, the proportion of adoptive placements with foster parents rose from 35% in SFY 1974, to 53% in SFY 1980, to 68% in 1985.[3] The impact of adoption subsidies, and federal participation in such programs, is clear.

REASONS FOR RELINQUISHMENT

Why would a mother relinquish her child for adoption? The answer to this question is complicated by the fact that, as we have just seen, the sources of children for adoption have been changing. Hardly any research exists concerning mothers in other countries who relinquish their children for foreign adoption, and the question might not even make sense in regard to mothers whose children have been more or less taken from them and sent on a convoluted route through foster care into adoption under the name of child protection and permanency planning.

Nonetheless, it will be instructive to review the research literature that does exist, keeping in mind that virtually all of it pertains to mothers who relinquished infants for domestic adoption before or during the 1960s and early 1970s, and that many of the research studies refer to white adolescent mothers who relinquished their children through private agencies.

Early research characterized unwed mothers who kept their children as more psychologically unstable than those who relinquished their children for adoption (Meyer et al., 1959; Yelloly, 1965). Later research found the relinquishers to be no more or less disturbed than those who kept their children (Grow, 1979). In any event, attributional studies do not address the question of "why" or "how" the decisions are made.

The factor that has been found to be most strongly and consistently associated with relinquishment is the influence of the unwed mother's parents. In a British study of adoption decision-making, the parents' unwillingness to accept the child into the family and desire that the child be adopted proved stronger than any other factor studied: in 51% of the cases in which the child was relinquished, the parents had this attitude, compared with only 10% of the cases in which the child was kept (Yelloly, 1965). In a New York City study, the factor most strongly associated with relinquishment was parental attitude: in none of the 67 cases studied in which the mother surrendered the child did the mother's parents approve of her keeping the child; conversely, parents' approval of keeping the child was detected from case records in regard to 42% of white mothers and 56% of black mothers who kept their children (Festinger, 1971). Not only was this the strongest association found in the study, but it was also one of the few associations found to be statistically significant for black as well as white mothers. In another New York City study, of 48 black and Puerto Rican pregnant adolescents, in every case in which the adolescent's mother planned to have the baby adopted, the adolescent agreed; and in 63% of the cases in which the adolescent's mother planned to keep the baby in the family home, the adolescent agreed (Young et al., 1975). A study of pregnant unwed adolescents in Michigan in 1974-1975 reported that 79% of those who decided to release their child for adoption reported that they had been influenced at least somewhat by their mother (50% said "a lot"), and the mother's influence was found to be greater than the father's (Rosen, 1980).

The role of parental influence in the decision-making process, which has received such consistent and strong support in what little research literature there is, can be viewed as a crucial factor that helps us to understand many of the other research findings. It would seem that the parents, and especially the mother, have been the key transmitters, at least up through the 1960s and early 1970s, of the then-prevailing cultural values against unwed motherhood and of the social stigmatization of that role.

These being the prevailing cultural values, social workers and other professionals at that time might have exerted influence in the same direction. In his study of the retrospective reports of 20 women who had relinquished a child for adoption (and who had become known to him as psychiatric outpatients), Rynearson (1982, p. 339) found: "All of the subjects perceived relinquishment as an externally enforced decision that overwhelmed their internal wish for continued attachment to the baby." Among the external factors he cited were "parental demands for relinquishment, social demands for parenthood only within marriage, and altruistic demands for the infant." In a questionnaire study of a narrow segment of relinquishers, those who were members of Concerned United Birthparents, a national organization formed in the 1970s, more than 300 respondents, the majority of whom apparently had relinquished during the 1960s, constituted the sample. The investigators found: "External factors, including family opposition, pressure from physicians or social workers, and financial constraints were cited by 69% of the sample as the primary reasons for surrender" (Deykin et al., 1984, p. 273). A study of 22 mothers who had surrendered a child for adoption years earlier and known to the investigators through their psychotherapy practice, yielded this finding: "Most reported that social workers and counselors offered no options, (and) emphasized instead that others could provide better lives for their children . . ." (Millen & Roll, 1985, p.415).

Other factors found to be significantly associated with the adoption decision included the following. The mother had other children and the putative father was married (Yelloly, 1965). The relinquishing mother tended to be younger, was more likely to be a student, and was less likely to be living independently than the nonrelinquishing mother. She was also less likely to have an ongoing relationship with the putative father, to have marriage plans, and to come from a broken home than the nonrelinquishing mother (Festinger, 1971). By the early 1970s, older women were more likely to relinquish than younger women, and the relinquishing mother was more likely to be living independently, less likely to report that the baby's father was supportive of her during pregnancy, and less likely to receive help during pregnancy from family and friends than the nonrelinquishing mother (Grow, 1979).

These findings can be seen as consistent with the centrality of the factors of parental influence and perceived availability of options. That is, a younger girl is less capable of even formulating plans on her own and is thus more subject to parental influence. She is also less capable of supporting herself, as is also true of a student, or a mother who has other children. If a relationship with the father is out of the question, this again limits options and subjects the girl more strongly to the influence of her parents. On the other hand, less influence is likely to be exerted by parents in a broken home than in a stable one. And if the girl is living with her parents, opportunity for parental influence is greater. By the early 1970s, however, overall relinquishments were declining, the social stigmatization of unwed motherhood was lessening, and perhaps parents were less inclined to exert influence toward adoption. Under these circumstances, it could be that young girls were less likely to relinquish because parents were supportive of them in the parents' home. Perhaps it would then more likely be the occasional older woman, living independently, and who did not have the support of parents, who would perceive few options other than to give her child up for adoption.

It has consistently been documented that blacks have been far less prone to relinquish children for adoption than whites (Festinger, 1971; Resnick, 1984), that the educational level of relinquishers has been greater than or no less than that of nonrelinquishers, and that the socioeconomic level of relinquishers has been higher or no lower than nonrelinquishers (Grow, 1979). Indeed, it seems that, especially during the 1960s, the social conventions against illegitimate childbirth and single parent motherhood were especially strong amongst the middle-class, and many middle-class girls were threatened with being "cut off" from their embarrassed parents if they did not relinquish the child for adoption. Not having anywhere else to turn, they succumbed to the influence of their parents and even internalized the prevailing social values against single parenthood. Thus an interview study of parents who had relinquished a child for adoption years earlier revealed that two-thirds gave as the reason for relinquishment that they were unmarried and wanted the child to have a family (Pannor et al., 1978).

Similar patterns of externally imposed limited options have been observed in New Zealand and Australia. Pressured by parents and social workers to give up her baby, the young pregnant girl was even kept ignorant of potential welfare benefits (Shawyer, 1979, p. 10). Self-reports of Australian women who relinquished children for adoption indicate a pattern of parental rejection, ostracism, social workers' pressure for a surrender decision and no alternatives or even information about alternatives offered (Inglis, 1984): "At no time did any person at all treat me as if I was a young mother in need of help" (p. 28). "How could you make plans in a place like that (at a home for girls in 'trouble') with no money and having to hide away? . . . Adoption was the way out everybody kept pointing me to. Somehow I knew it wasn't, but I didn't know anything else" (pp.34-35). "The nun's attitude was that adoption was the best thing to do for the baby; you had to think of the baby, not yourself . . . (My parents) never discussed the possibility of me keeping the baby" (pp. 55,64).

POVERTY AND ADOPTION

As already noted, the foregoing research studies pertained to relinquishments of infants for domestic adoption, mostly before or during the 1960s and early 1970s, and often by white adolescent mothers through private agencies. These characteristics did accurately reflect the population of relinquishers and adoptions at that time, and so the findings in regard to the reasons and factors related to relinquishment are valid for that time. Currently, however, we can estimate that the majority of nonrelated adoptions, perhaps 53% and rising, are a combination of adoptions of children coming from the public agency foster care system, and foreign adoptions.

This still leaves a sizable percentage of independent and private agency adoptions, other than foreign adoptions. But we cannot automatically assume that the smaller number of American mothers who release infants for private agency and independent adoption in the 1980s do so for the same reasons that their counterparts did in the 1960s and early 1970s.

In the 1980s, single parent families are commonplace, and normative conventions against unwed mothers have eroded considerably. Abortion is widely used as a form of birth control when unwanted pregnancy is not prevented by contraception. Moreover, beyond these options, far larger numbers of single teenage mothers than in the past feel free to, and do, raise their own children. Many remain in their parents' home, and many others live independently. They avail themselves of public assistance, or find work to support themselves, and increased social services are available to them.

In this current transformed social context, with greatly expanded alternatives, it cannot be assumed that parental influence in the direction of adoption continues to be a major factor in the adoption decision, but merely amongst a smaller subset of our society. And yet again it might be. We simply do not know, and this is a matter for further investigation.

Clues are available, however, in regard to factors related to relinquishment in the growth sector of nonrelated adoptions: foreign adoptions, and the adoption of children coming out of our public foster care system.

As already indicated, the greatest source of foreign adoptions into the United States continues to be South Korea. It is remarkable that in 1985, more than 30 years after the Korean War, South Korea relinquished more children for adoption in the United States than in any previous year.

Up until the mid-1960s, most children relinquished in South Korea for foreign adoption were of mixed race, having been fathered by American soldiers. Such children had been severely ostracized in Korean society, to an extent that was reason enough for their mothers to relinquish them for adoption abroad. As far back as 1973, however, 97% of Korean-born children adopted by foreigners were "pure" Koreans (Kim, 1978). Why would such children be given up for adoption?

There has been a traditionally strong emphasis in Korea on family blood ties, and a severe social stigmatization of "illegitimate" children and their mothers (Kim, 1978). Yet a study of Korean parents whose children were adopted abroad (summarized by Kim, 1978) shows that one-third of the 98 children in the study were born to parents who were in common-law relationships, and 30% were born legitimate. About one-fifth (presumably composed of those who were born legitimate) had parents who were married to each other at the time of relinquishment (Kim, 1978). The most frequent reason for relinquishment appearing in the case records and given by agency social workers was "illegitimacy." However, "no capacity to raise" and "poverty, failure in family planning, too many children" were also frequent reasons. Moreover, it was determined that the natural fathers in the cases studied had low-income jobs, and most of the natural mothers were either unemployed or had low-paying jobs such as waitress, bus-girl, housemaid, or factory worker. The researcher concluded that lack of financial capacity to raise the children was a major cause of relinquishment. However, it seems that this was one of several related factors, including the social stigmatization of illegitimacy and pressure from extended family members, that combined to restrict the mothers' alternatives (Kim, 1978). Indeed, such external factors probably served to cut off economic and social support thus forcing the adoption decision.

If a South Korean mother is living in poverty, not much assistance is likely to come from the government. In 1981, less than 1% of the South Korean government budget went for all social welfare programs combined, and prior to that year, mothers with dependent children were ineligible for any government assistance, although it was established at that time that over one million children needed assistance (Alstein, 1984). According to one observer who visited child welfare personnel in Korea: "Extreme poverty, an ever-increasing population, and the government's inability to provide adequately for abandoned children are the main reasons Korea is one of the 'prime exporters' of children" (Alstein, 1984, p.201).

Between 1945 and 1980, South Korea's urban population grew from 15% to 57% of the total population, mostly as a result of migration from rural areas (Seekins, 1982). The city of Seoul grew from under one million to more than six million during those years (Lee, 1980). Many commentators attribute to such change, in South Korea as well as other countries, the breakdown of stable extended family structures that were present in rural society, as people migrate to and fail to find jobs in the cities, or otherwise remain poor, and hence the increasing abandonment of children (e.g., Baig & Gopinath, 1976; Benet, 1976, pp. 121-122; Goriawalla, 1976; Joe, 1978; Kim, 1978; and Goldschmidt, 1986).

In Colombia, too, there has been a high rate of rural to urban migration since the 1940s, resulting in a deterioration of kinship ties. Agricultural workers leave the rural areas hoping to improve their way of life, but being uneducated and unskilled, they merely exchange rural poverty for urban poverty. The continued flood of this migration has made it difficult for men to find even the most menial jobs, and there is a high rate of unemployment and underemployment in this migrant population, although women often find jobs as domestic servants or cooks. Many of the migrants become residents of the shantytowns that surround the larger cities (Blutstein et al., 1977, pp. 93, 115). Moreover, among this population:

> Formal marriage is frequently not the basis of the family or household, and the father is sometimes not a permanent member of the family circle. Children may be fathered in a series of free unions in which men move in temporarily with the mother. (Blutstein et al., 1977, p. 118)

Social security benefits in Colombia are available only to those who are or were employed, and their dependents (Blutstein et al., 1977, pp. 195-197; Resnick & Rodriguez, 1982). However, agricultural, domestic, and temporary workers receive few benefits, and even for those entitled, the typical social security payment per child was less than two dollars per month in 1973 (Resnick & Rodriguez, 1982). By the mid-1970s, the Colombian government was administering day care services for only 13,500 children, although five million children were in need of such services (Resnick and Rodriguez, 1982).

A survey of Colombian agency professional staff, judges, lawyers, health professionals, and other Colombians who deal with adoptions revealed that almost all (89%) believed that economic pressure was frequently the reason that Colombian parents abandon their children or release them for adoption (Resnick & Rodriguez, 1982). Half also thought that abandonment by spouse or companion was frequently the reason, and slightly less than half believed that social pressures or rejection (of single motherhood) was frequently the reason. Less than one-third (30%) thought that personality traits or immaturity were frequently the reason.

A survey of 46 families who had adopted Colombian children revealed that 24% of the children required hospitalization or extensive medical treatment at the time of their adoption or shortly thereafter, most often due to poverty, inadequate nutrition, and poor medical care available in Colombia (Feigelman & Silverman, 1983, p.139). Indeed, a 1973 study found that two-thirds of all five-year-old children in Colombia suffered from some degree of malnutrition, and that each year malnutrition caused the deaths of 30,000 children (Blutstein et al., 1977, p. 189). Of course, this situation is not limited to Colombia. Through a questionnaire sent to hundreds of couples in the Netherlands who had adopted a foreign child, it was found that 20% of the children were reported by the adoptive parents to have been suffering from some degree of malnutrition when received, 15% from intestinal disorders, and 15% from various forms of skin disease. Nearly 30% exhibited an almost insatiable craving for food (Hoksbergen, 1981).

In Colombia, street children roam the large cities (Joe, 1978; Goldschmidt, 1986). In Brazil, millions of abandoned and needy children are growing up in the city streets. Seven million Brazilian children have lost all or most links with their families. More than half of Brazilian children under the age of six years old are undernourished. Family disintegration in Brazil is due to large-scale peasant migration from the impoverished northeast to urban slums in the south (Riding, 1985). Speaking of Latin America in general, Goldschmidt (1986, p.261) comments: "Because there is insufficient protection for mothers and too few measures to strengthen the family, women who are left on their own are often forced to abandon their children for economic reasons."

Indian commentators have likewise attributed the abandonment of children in their country to urbanization, together with lack of supportive services from the government to meet the needs brought about by the break-up of extended families (Baig & Gopinath, 1976; Sohoni, 1976). In India in 1971, 46 million of its 228 million children under 14 years were estimated to be living below the poverty level (Baig & Gopinath, 1976). In India, too, social stigmatization of the unmarried mother and the "illegitimate" child plays a role (Goriawalla, 1976; Kulkarni, 1976).

We see that two factors keep cropping up in relation to adoption: poverty and "illegitimacy." Either alone or together, they are not sufficient to cause the relinquishment of children for adoption. *Relinquishment occurs when the poverty of rural areas is exchanged for the poverty of urban areas, where there is a concomitant severance of external sources of support for the mother and child. Relinquishment is also more likely to occur when unwed mothers are socially ostracized, because this again cuts off external sources of support.*

In societies in which unwed motherhood is socially stigmatized, this stigmatization is likely to affect government welfare policy, so that public aid will not be extended to unwed mothers, leaving them in poverty and without support. In the United States, there was a time when "illegitimacy" was severely stigmatized. Young unwed mothers were threatened with isolation from their own parents if they did not relinquish their infants for adoption. They could have turned to public aid, and perhaps many did, because in the United States the stigmatization did not totally invade public policy (although locally established "suitable home" criteria that excluded "illegitimate" children were invoked for a time; see Bell, 1965). But perhaps the threatened cut-off of social support, ignorance of public aid, and the prospect of a greatly reduced material level of living were enough to frighten many young unwed mothers into relinquishing their children. They were not encouraged to understand that alternatives existed.

Although illegitimate births can certainly occur among middle-class women, poverty is related to "illegitimacy" in several ways. First, urban poverty creates the social conditions that cause births to be "illegitimate." Women who do not have their own resources are subject to the whims of men. If men, because of their own job instability, walk in and out of their lives without marrying them, then they are subject to "illegitimate" births. Second, where "illegitimacy" is stigmatized, it can cause poverty among young women by cutting them off from the financial support of their own parents and community. Third, where "illegitimacy" is stigma-

tized, it can cause the unavailability of public economic aid to unwed mothers, due to designation of such mothers as among the
"unworthy poor" in social policy.

*The most prevalent and general causes of relinquishment of chil-
dren for adoption, then, are that the mother is or faces the prospect
of living in poverty, is or faces the prospect of being cut off from
previous family supports, and new sources of support are not available or not sought.* In this general form, these principles apply
equally as well to the American mothers who relinquished children
for adoption back in the 1960s, as they do to foreign adoptions
today.

No wonder, then, that the low number of Swedish children available for adoption has been attributed to relative lack of discrimination against women in the job market, the absence of stigmatization
of the unmarried mother, and governmental economic and social
supports for mothers (Benet, 1976, pp. 92-93). On the other hand,
where poverty is found, due to sex discrimination or any other factors, and where supports are not available to offset it, the relinquishment of children is fostered.

On the one side are the pressures of poverty. On the other is the
narrow range of alternatives imposed and structured by others,
namely, support for the child only under condition that the mother
allow the child to be permanently separated from her. The mother's
response options are limited to watching her child starve, or relinquishing all rights to the child, never to see him or her again. In
South Korea, as in other countries, the only recourse for some
mothers was to abandon the child to an institution (Benet, 1976,
pp. 124-125).

The clearest documentation of the flow of *domestically* adopted
children from indigent parents to those who are economically better
off is found in Israel. Data available on domestic adoptions for the
period 1970-1977 in Israel indicate that 71% of the children adopted
by nonrelatives were relinquished by Sephardi mothers, while most
adoptive parents were Ashkenazi (Jaffe, 1982, pp. 202-203). The
socioeconomic significance of this fact is that in 1975-1976, 56% of
the families in the lowest net income decile in Israel were Sephardi
Jews (that is, of Asian and African background) while only 6% of
families in the highest decile were Sephardi. In contrast, 70% of the

families in the highest income decile were Ashkenazi (of European and American background), while only 11% of the families in the lowest decile were Ashkenazi (Jaffe, 1982, pp. 83-84).

What makes the situation in Israel especially interesting is that the Sephardi Jews tend to be of darker skin complexion than Ashkenazi Jews. The fact that the Sephardis, like the Ashkenazis, are Jews, apparently has overridden, in many cases, any reluctance to adopt due to darker skin. Blacks in American society have held a comparable economic position to that of Sephardis in Israeli Jewish society. Yet in the United States, for a variety of reasons, few black children had been adopted in the past. This fact contributed to a weak relationship between adoption and prior poverty of the natural mother in the United States. In Israel, however, the relationship between poverty and adoption has been clearly visible.

In capsule form, in Israeli society, we see a similar pattern of adoption flow that is going on in the world at large today in regard to foreign adoptions: from the disadvantaged to the advantaged. It was the dwindling of the supply of white infants for adoption in the United States and the European countries that led to a turn toward Third World countries, particularly in Asia and Latin America, for children to adopt. While this has necessitated looking to children of darker skin complexion (oriental children and, in the case of Latin American countries, children of mixed European and Indian origin), very few children come from Africa. As we have seen however, due to the permanency planning movement in the United States, increasing numbers of American black children are now being adopted.

The source of children for adoption through the permanency planning movement is foster care, and we know that most of the children in the foster care system were placed there from impoverished families. For example, in a study of children in foster care in New York City, it was found that 52% of the families from which the children came had been receiving some form of public assistance at the time of placement (Jenkins & Norman, 1972). The authors observed that just prior to placement, "most of the children in the study lived in impoverished households located in the poorest neighborhoods" (p.19) of that city. In a study of children in foster care in Massachusetts, it was found that in 1972, 60% of the biological families had incomes of less than $5,000 per year, and 37%

even received less than $3,000. Forty percent of the families were receiving public assistance (Gruber, 1978).

In New Jersey, case record analysis of a sample of children who entered foster care in 1971 revealed that no one in the natural family was employed in 68% of the cases (Claburn & Magura, 1977). A study of children placed in foster care in New Jersey during 1977 showed that 60% of the natural families had annual incomes of under $5,000, and 56% were receiving some form of public assistance (Levit, 1979). This study also indicated that the general economic status of the natural families of children in foster family care is lower than that of the families of children in residential-institutional care, when foster care is divided into these two subgroups. (The far larger proportion of children are in foster family care and most children are adopted from this subgroup [Fein & Maluccio, 1984].) Eighty percent of the natural families of children in foster family care had annual incomes of under $5,000, and less than 1% had incomes above $10,000 per year. Sixty-eight percent were receiving some form of public assistance.

Jenkins and Norman (1972, p. 19) state in regard to foster care:

> For most households poverty is a necessary but not a sufficient condition for placement. It is the marginal family, whose characteristics and social circumstances are such that it cannot sustain further stress, which utilizes the placement system as a last resort when its own fragile support systems break down.

Indeed, a study of a sample of almost 700 case records of children who entered foster care in New Jersey during the first three-quarters of 1983 revealed that homelessness was the precipitating reason for placement in 14% of the cases, and that altogether, the families of 40% of the children had at some time experienced homelessness or severe housing difficulties (Tomaszewicz, 1985). In 1984, inadequate housing was the most prevalent reason for foster care placement in New Jersey, accounting for 15% of the children residing in foster care at that time (New Jersey State Child Placement Advisory Council, 1984).

Other reasons for placement frequently identified in studies of foster care, usually based on caseworkers' judgments, include "parent unable to cope," child neglect, abandonment, child abuse, child's behavioral problems, parent's drug or alcohol abuse, parent's physical illness, and "hospitalization" (New Jersey State Child Placement Advisory Council, 1984[5]). However, if poverty does not constitute a "sufficient condition" for placement, neither do the "reasons" cited in the foster care studies. For example, the mother's illness or hospitalization cannot be sufficient reason, since there are many mothers similarly indisposed whose children are *not* placed. Even alleged child abuse or neglect is not sufficient reason for placement, since many children who have been abused or neglected in the past can be served and protected in their own homes. The strong relationship that has consistently been found between alleged child abuse and neglect and poverty (Pelton, 1978) suggests that the problem most often is the parent's lack of ability to cope with poverty and its stresses without help (Pelton, 1978, 1982). The more accurate reason for placement is very often that the family, often due to poverty, does not have the resources to offset the impact of situational or personal problems, which themselves are often caused by poverty, *and the agencies have failed to provide the needed supports*. Most children in foster care are there because their parents were unable, or did not have the personal resources, to overcome family crises without additional outside assistance, which was not forthcoming.

The foregoing analysis, then, provides a description of the needs and circumstances of the pool of families and their children in foster care from which the permanency planning policy is currently extracting children for adoption. The direct link between poverty, adoption, and lack of preventive support is illustrated, for example, by the fact that in New York City in 1981, adoption was the discharge objective for 29% of the children for whom inadequate housing had been at least one of the reasons for placement in foster care, and for 32% of the children for whom inadequate finances had been one of the reasons.[5]

CONCLUSIONS AND IMPLICATIONS

Throughout most of the 20th century, the stated commitment of American child welfare policy has been to preserve families. The tone was set by the proclamation of the 1909 White House Conference on the Care of Dependent Children that children "should as a rule be kept with their parents, such aid being given as may be necessary to maintain suitable homes for the rearing of the children" and that "except in unusual circumstances, the home should not be broken up for reasons of poverty" (Bremner, 1971, p. 365). This commitment has been reinforced by the "reasonable efforts" clause of the AACWA of 1980.

When homelessness and poverty figure so prominently among the exceptions to the rule, we must wonder whether the policy cannot be more diligently implemented. Ironically, as we have seen, the permanency planning provisions of the AACWA have given a boost to the most extreme form of severance of parental ties for many children. This might not be a cause for concern if we could be confident that all reasonable efforts are being made to prevent the separation of children from parents in the first instance.

Surely, once children have been broken from their families for whatever faults or shortcomings of their country's economy or social system, or of their government's provisions for those in need, there is nothing inhumane about others taking it upon themselves to care for such children. But the humane response of individual adoptive parents to children in need of care is preceded by an inhumane collective response to the needs of destitute families that first denies them necessary resources, and then offers only an extreme alternative. At present, the entire public and professional discourse on adoption is marked by a glaring unconcern with the "front end" of the institution of adoption, with the parents who give birth to the children, and the circumstances that cause them to relinquish their children.

The humane care given to adopted children by adoptive parents comes after the fact — the fact that reasonable efforts were not made to prevent the need for separating children from their natural parents, whether we speak of children being adopted from foreign countries, or children being adopted within our own country out of the foster care system.

Collectively, efforts must be redoubled to implement the stated child welfare policy of preserving families. Insofar as possible, this policy should be applied to concern for children in foreign countries as well as in the United States. The child welfare establishment and social work profession should intensify their concerns with international child welfare and focus on the prevention of the need to separate children from parents. They have the obligation to research more fully the sources of foreign adoptions, and to contribute, to the shaping of American foreign policy in a direction which includes a greater focus on child and family welfare in other countries.

NOTES

1. Immigration and Naturalization Service, Statistical Analysis Branch. Table IMM 2.5. Immigrant orphans admitted to the United States by country or region of birth: Fiscal years 1981-1985.

2. Pelton, L. H. (1986). Whose neglect? The role of poverty-related factors in child neglect cases and court decisions. Unpublished manuscript.

3. Adoption placement statistics for 1963-1985 for New Jersey were provided (in the form of tables) to the author by Mary Lou Sweeney, Supervisor of the Central Office Adoption Unit, New Jersey Division of Youth and Family Services, Trenton, NJ.

4. Annual adoption placement statistical reports for state fiscal years 1970-1985 for Tennessee were provided to the author by Joyce N. Harris, Program Manager, Adoptions, Tennessee Department of Human Services, Nashville, TN.

5. CWIS/CCRS Special Report Series, New York City, Series A, Status date 3/31/81. P. 6, Table 13, and pp. 36-37, Table 34.

REFERENCES

Adams, J. E. & Kim, H. B. (1971). A fresh look at intercountry adoptions. *Children*, *18*, 214-221.

Alstein, H. (1984). Transracial and intercountry adoptions: A comparison. In P. Sachdev (Ed.), *Adoption: Current issues and trends* (pp. 195-203). Toronto, Canada: Butterworths.

Bachrach, C. A. (1986). Adoption plans, adopted children, and adoptive mothers. *Journal of Marriage and the Family*, *48*, 243-253.

Baig, T. A. & Gopinath, C. (1976). Adoption—The Indian scene. *Indian Journal of Social Work*, *37*, 135-140.

Bell, W. (1965). *Aid to dependent children*. New York: Columbia University Press.

Benet, M.K. (1976). *The politics of adoption*. New York: Free Press.

Blutstein, H. I., Edwards, J.D., Johnston, K. T., Mc Morris, D. S. & Rudolph, J. D. (1977). *Area handbook for Colombia* (3rd ed.) Washington, D.C.: U. S. Government Printing Office.

Bonham, G. S. (1977). Who adopts: The relationship of adoption and social-demographic characteristics of women. *Journal of Marriage and the Family*, *39*, 295-306.

Bremner, R. H. (Ed.) (1971). *Children and youth in America: A documentary history* (Vol. 2). Cambridge, MA: Harvard University Press.

Claburn, W. E. & Magura, S. (1977). *Foster care review in New Jersey: An evaluation of its implementation and effects*. Final report (Federal grant no. 18-p-90275/2-01). Social and Rehabilitation Services, U. S. Department of Health, Education and Welfare.

Deykin, E. Y., Campbell, L. & Patti, P. (1984). The postadoption experience of surrendering parents. *American Journal of Orthopsychiatry*, *57*, 271-280.

Emlen, A., Lahti, J., Downs, G., McKay, A. & Downs, S. (1978). *Overcoming barriers to planning for children in foster care*. Washington, DC: DHEW Publication No. (OHDS) 78-30138.

Fanshel, D. & Shinn, E. B. (1978). *Children in foster care: A longitudinal investigation.* New York: Columbia University Press.

Feigelman, W. & Silverman, A. R. (1983). *Chosen children*. New York: Praeger.

Fein, E. & Maluccio, A. (1984). Children leaving foster care: Outcomes of permanency planning. *Child Abuse and Neglect, 8*, 425-431.

Festinger, T. B. (1971). Unwed mothers and their decisions to keep or surrender children. *Child Welfare, 50*, 253-263.

Fopp, P. (1982). Inter-country adoption: Australia's position. *Australian Journal of Social Issues, 17*, 50-61.

Goldschmidt, I. (1986). National and intercountry adoptions in Latin America. *International Social Work, 29*, 257-268.

Goriawalla, N. M. (1976). Inter-country adoptions – Policy and practice with reference to India. *Indian Journal of Social Work, 37*, 151-158.

Grow, L. J. (1979). Today's unmarried mothers: The choices have changed. *Child Welfare, 58*, 363-371.

Gruber, A. R. (1978). *Children in foster care: Destitute, neglected – betrayed*. New York: Human Sciences Press.

Hoksbergen, R. A. C. (1981). Adoption of foreign children in the Netherlands. *International Child Welfare Review, 49*, 26-37.

Immigration and Naturalization Service. 1980 statistical yearbook of the Immigration and Naturalization Service. Washington, DC: U.S. Department of Justice.

Inglis, K. (1984). *Living mistakes*. Sydney, Australia: George Allen & Unwin.

Jaffe, E. D. (1982). *Child welfare in Israel*. New York: Praeger.

Jenkins, S. & Norman, E. (1972). *Fillial deprivation and foster care*. New York: Columbia University Press.

Joe, B. (1978). In defense of intercountry adoption. *Social Service Review, 52*, 1-20.

Kim, D. S. (1978). From women to women with painful love: A study of maternal motivation in intercountry adoption process. In H. H. Sunoo & D. S. Kim (Eds), *Korean women in a struggle for humanization* (pp. 117-169). Memphis, TN: Association of Korean Christian Scholars in North America.

Knitzer, J., Allen, M. L. & Mc Gowan, B. (1978). *Children without homes: An examination of public responsibility to children in out-of-home care*. Washington, DC: Children's Defense Fund.

Krichefsky, G. D. (1961). Alien orphans. *I & N Reporter* (U. S. Department of Justice, Immigration and Naturalization Service), *9*, 43-51.

Kulkarni, A. (1976). Adoption and foster care – Domestic and international. *Indian Journal of Social Work, 37*, 165-170.

Lee, M. G. (1980). Characteristics of social change. In S. Park, T. Shin & K. Z. O. (Eds.), *Economic development and social change in Korea* (pp. 273-287). Frankfurt, Germany: Campus-Verlag.

Levit, L. D. (1979). *Characteristics of DYFS children in residential and foster care*. Trenton, NJ: Division of Budget and Program Review, Office of Legislative Services, New Jersey State Legislature.

Maas, H. S. (1969). Children in long-term foster care. *Child Welfare, 48*, 321-333.

Maas, H. S. & Engler, Jr., R. E. (1959). *Children in need of parents*. New York: Columbia University Press.

Maza, P. L. (1984). Adoption trends: 1944-1975. *Child Welfare Research Notes, #9*, August. Administration for Children, Youth, and Families, U.S. Department of Health and Human Services.

Meyer, H. J., Borgatta, E. F. & Fanshel, D. (1959). Unwed mothers' decisions about their babies: An interim replication report. *Child Welfare, 38*, 1-6.

Millen, L. & Roll, S. (1985). Solomon's mothers: A special case of pathological bereavement. *American Journal of Orthopsychiatry, 55*, 411-418.

National Center for Social Statistics. (1973). *Adoptions in 1971*. Washington, DC: U.S. Department of Health, Education, and Welfare.

National Center for Social Statistics. (1975). *Adoptions in 1973*. Washington, DC: U.S. Department of Health, Education, and Welfare.

National Center for Social Statistics. (1976). *Adoptions in 1974*. Washington, DC: U.S. Department of Health, Education, and Welfare.

National Committee for Adoption. (1985). *Adoption factbook: United States data, issues, regulations, and resources*. Washington, DC: Author.

New Jersey State Child Placement Advisory Council (1984). *New Jersey Judiciary 1984 report on child placement review*. Trenton, NJ: Administrative Office of the Courts.

Pannor, R., Baran, A. & Sorosky, A. D. (1978). Birth parents who relinquished babies for adoption revisited. *Family Process, 17*, 329-337.

Pelton, L. H. (1978). Child abuse and neglect: The myth of classlessness. *American Journal of Orthopsychiatry, 48*, 608-617.

Pelton, L. H. (1982). Personalistic attributions and client perspectives in child welfare cases: Implications for service delivery. In T. A. Wills (Ed.), *Basic processes in helping relationships* (pp. 81-101). New York: Academic Press.

Pelton, L. H. (1987). Not for poverty alone: Foster care population trends in the twentieth century. *Journal of Sociology and Social Welfare*, in press.

Pilotti, F. J. (1985). Intercountry adoption: A view from Latin America. *Child Welfare, 64*, 25-35.

Resnick, M. D. (1984). Studying adolescent mothers' decision-making about adoption and parenting. *Social Work, 29*, 5-10.

Resnick, R. P. & Rodriguez, G. M. (1982). *Intercountry adoptions between the United States and Colombia*. New York: International Social Service.

Riding, A. (1985). Brazil's time bomb: Poor children by the millions. *New York Times*, October 23.

Rosen, R. H. (1980). Adolescent pregnancy decision-making: Are parents important? *Adolescence, 40*, 43-54.

Rynearson, E. K. (1982). Relinquishment and its maternal complications: A preliminary study. *American Journal of Psychiatry, 139*, 338-340.

Seekins, D. M. (1982). The society and its environment. In F. M. Bunge (Ed.), *South Korea: A country study* (3rd ed., pp. 49-105). Washington, DC: U.S. Government Printing Office.

Shawyer, J. (1979). *Death by adoption*. Auckland, New Zealand: Cicada Press.

Shyne, A. W. & Schroeder, A. G. (1978). *National study of social services to children and their families: Overview*. Washington, DC: U.S. Department of Health, Education, and Welfare.

Sohoni, N. K. (1976). Role of adoption and foster care in child rehabilitation. *Indian Journal of Social Work, 37*, 121-134.

Stein, T. J. & Gambrill, E. D. (1985). Permanency planning for children: The past and present. *Children and Youth Services Review, 7*, 83-94.

Tatara, T. & Pettiford, E.K. (1985). *Characteristics of children in substitute and adoptive care*. Washington, DC: Voluntary Cooperative Information System, American Public Welfare Association.

Testa, M. & Lawlor, E. (1985). *The state of the child: 1985*. Chicago: The Chapin Hall Center for Children at the University of Chicago.

Tomaszewicz, M. C. (1985). *Children entering foster care: Factors leading to placement*. Trenton, NJ: New Jersey Division of Youth and Family Services.

Wald, M. S. (1976). State intervention on behalf of "neglected" children: Standards for removal from their homes, monitoring the status of children in foster care, and termination of parental rights. *Stanford Law Review, 28*, 623-706.

Weil, R. H. (1984). International adoptions: The quiet migration. *International Migration Review, 43*, 276-293.

Yelloly, M. A. (1965). Factors relating to an adoption decision by the mothers of illegitimate infants. *Sociological Review*, New Series, *13*, 5-14.

Young, A. T., Berkman, B. & Rehr, H. (1975). Parental influence on pregnant adolescents. *Social Work, 20*, 387-391.

Open Adoptions:
Practice and Policy Issues

Ruth G. McRoy
Harold D. Grotevant

SUMMARY. This article provides an overview of the controversy surrounding openness in adoptions practice and discusses the open options which many adoption agencies are currently offering adoptive and birth parents. The findings of an exploratory study which examine the impact of traditional, semi-open and fully-disclosed adoptions on adoptive and birth parents are presented. The risks and benefits of each type of adoption are described and policy and practice implications are discussed.

There has been much speculation on the subject of adoption, but very little examination of longer-term adjustment issues (McRoy, Grotevant & Zurcher, 1986; McRoy & Zurcher, 1983) and of adoptive family relationships (Kirk, 1959, 1964, 1981). During the past decade, there has been a growing debate over the issue of confidentiality in adoptions versus adoptees' rights to know their birthparents (Campbell, 1979; Cliff, 1983; Harrington, 1979; Foster, 1979; Sanders & Sitterly, 1981). Traditionally, social workers in the United States have insisted on closed records. That is, birthmothers and adoptive parents generally received limited demographic information about each other although adoptive parents may be given some medical background information. However, once relinquishment papers were signed, the birthmother would never see the child again and often would never know about the future of the child she placed for adoption. It was assumed that the birthmother wanted to maintain anonymity and wanted to forget she ever had given birth to the child. It was also assumed that this closed approach would facilitate relinquishment of the child both emotionally and legally (Kraft, Palombo, Mitchell, Woods, Schmidt & Tucker, 1985).

Similarly, the adoption agency has traditionally given the adoptive parents sketchy information on the birthparents of the child they adopted. Agency workers assumed that the attachment between the adoptive parents and the child would be better achieved if the parents felt secure in the permanence of the relationship and did not have to dwell on information about the birthparents. Generally, once the adoption was finalized, the agency had no further contact with the birthparents and therefore received no updated information on the birthparents' lives.

The policy which mandated confidentiality in adoptions was based upon the following assumed needs: the need for anonymity of parties involved in adoption; the need for completely severing the adoptee's ties to birthparents; the stigma of illegitimacy; and the assumption that normal, well-adjusted individuals would-and-should—know only the parents who raised them (Kraft, et al., 1985). Generally, the agency social worker made decisions regarding what specific information should be shared with the adoptive parents. It was assumed that the adoptive parents would share this information with the child when they felt it was appropriate. Very rarely was additional information shared between the two parties.

However, recent research findings on relinquishing mothers have revealed that many birthmothers still experience symptoms of mourning at the anniversary of the relinquishment, although the intensity of the mourning responses diminished with time (Rynearson, 1982). Many birthmothers may wonder whether they made the right decision to place, if the child is still alive, how the child feels about them, or if the child has a good home. This process is especially complex for adolescent birthmothers, whose cognitive and emotional immaturity may exacerbate their reactions to pregnancy and relinquishment of parental rights.

Many researchers and clinicians agree that adopted children lack adequate knowledge about their birthparents as well (Brinich, 1980; Colon, 1978; Sorosky, Baran & Pannor, 1975, 1984; Triseliotis, 1973). Adoptees appear to be more vulnerable to identity problems developing in adolescence than are their nonadopted peers (Sorosky et al., 1975). They may wonder about their birthmothers' reasons for relinquishing them for adoption. Some may feel that their birthparents rejected them. Others may fantasize about the whereabouts of their first set of parents and wish to find them, and others who have no knowledge of their birthparents have no interest in learning about their backgrounds (Sorosky et al., 1984).

Under the traditional closed adoptions process, adoptive parents are faced with the task of answering the adoptees' questions with very limited information, adopted children know little about their genealogical background, and birthparents have very little if any information about the fate of their child. In the early 1970s, as more and more adoptees and birthparents returned to the agency to seek additional background information, some agencies began offering relinquishing birthmothers and prospective adoptive families a continuum of openness which is dependent on the needs and desires of the members of the adoption triad. Birthparents and adopting parents could choose among the following options: to exchange nonidentifying information; to know first names only; to meet without identifying themselves; to meet with full disclosure of names and addresses; to exchange letters, pictures, or phone calls; and/or to have sustained contact (Children's Home Society of California, 1984).

Agency workers believed that these open options might help birthparents feel less pain and guilt, ease adoptive parents' fear and questions, provide adoptees with biological continuity, and "humanize" the adoption process (Sorich & Siebert, 1982). Moreover, advocates of open adoption believe that knowledge of one's past is a basic human need and emotional problems may result when this knowledge is denied (Curtis, 1986).

Since their inception these practices have been very controversial. Some proponents suggest that adoption is generally a second choice option for infertile parents, and that through the traditional closed adoption procedure they can pretend that "the adopted child was, in fact, born to them" (Pannor & Baran, 1984, p. 248). Advocates of openness believe that adoptive and birthparents should routinely meet and exchange identifying information so that adoptive parents cannot deny the adoption, birthparents can better cope with feelings of mourning and grief, and adoptees can gain a more realistic understanding of their birthparents' reasons for relinquishing (Pannor & Baran, 1984). Opponents suggest that open adoption violates the privacy of adoptive parents and birthparents alike and would confuse the adopted child with the introduction of multiple parents (Foster, 1979; Kraft et al., 1985; Zeilinger, 1979). Until now, the arguments pro and con were heavily value laden and lacked any empirical evidence concerning the impact on the adoption triad. This paper presents the findings of a small exploratory study which was designed to begin to identify some of the issues and consequences of open adoptions.

AN EXPLORATORY STUDY OF OPENNESS IN ADOPTION

In the Fall of 1984, Lutheran Social Service of Texas (LSS) commissioned an exploratory study which would evaluate the consequences of openness in adoption as practiced by three regional offices of the agency (McRoy, Grotevant & White, 1985). In 1977, the agency had begun educating adoptive couples on openness issues and helped them consider some communication with the birthparent. The procedure began with the exchange of one letter and later ongoing correspondence. New options became available as birthparents, adoptive parents and adopted individuals expressed their needs, frustrations and hopes as they have assumed their roles in the adoption triad. These included an exchange of first names; ongoing correspondence through the agency; and exchange of pictures and gifts. Beginning in the Summer of 1981, the San Antonio and Corpus Christi offices of LSS began a pilot project in which they offered an additional form of openness of prospective parents and birthparents: face-to-face meetings. Initially, these meetings were taped or monitored by a social worker. As they became more routine, monitoring ceased and adoptive parents and birthparents were allowed to share whatever they wished. Some chose to share identifying information and a few chose to have ongoing contact.

In order to assess the LSS families' experiences with these open options, 17 adoptive families and their corresponding birthparents were randomly selected for study participation from a listing of adoptive parents and birthparents provided by the regional offices.

Fifteen of the 17 corresponding birthparents agreed to participate in the study. Fourteen birthmothers, and one birthfather were interviewed individually. A birthgrandmother of one of the adopted children was also interviewed. At the time of the study, the children ranged in age from four months to six years of age. Therefore, the children themselves were not interviewed.

The adoptive sample consisted of 15 Anglo and two Hispanic couples. All the adoptive families were middle to upper-middle class based on family income. The adoptive mothers ranged in age from 31 to 42 years, the adoptive fathers from 30 to 47 years. Birthparent ages (at the time of the birth of their child) ranged from 14 to 42 years of age. Two birthparents were Hispanic and the remainder Anglo.

Data were collected by using a separate, semi-structured interview for the adoptive parents and birthparents. Interviews were held in an LSS office with 15 of the adoptive couples. In two cases, the adoptive parents were interviewed in their homes. Telephone interviews were conducted with three birthparents because they lived out of state. The remainder were interviewed in an LSS office. All of the interviews were audiotaped and transcribed. Questions focused on the degree of openness offered and selected by the adoptive and birthparents; reasons for choosing the option; perceived advantages and disadvantages of varying degrees of openness; satisfactions encountered; and perceived impact on the adoption triad.

The families were divided into three groups based on the degree of openness in their adoption. The first group included two families with *traditional adoptions*. There was little or no information shared between the adoptive and birthparents and no ongoing contact of any kind was present. When an attempt was made to contact the birthmothers for participation in this study, no response was received. The second group, five families with *semi-open adoptions*, had exchanged such item as pictures, gifts, or letters with birthparents. In one case, a fac o-face meeting had taken place, but no identifying information was shared and no ongoing contact was maintained. The third group, ten families with *fully-disclosed adoptions*, had disclosed identifying information and had ongoing contact between adoptive and birthparents and the children.

Families with Traditional Adoptions

Neither of the traditional adoptive families had been offered a choice about the degree of openness in the adoption, and they strongly indicated that they preferred having a traditional adoption. Both feared that the birthmother might take the child back (and that the courts might cooperate in this) if she had any contact with the child. They indicated that openness would be confusing to the child, especially when he or she was young. They also felt that they did not want anyone "looking over your shoulder" once the adoption was finalized. However, they did acknowledge that in traditional adoption, the adopted child might find it harder to locate a birthparent if he or she searches.

When asked about the potential advantages of open adoption, both families felt that there were few. The only advantages were seen to be for the child, and only when the child was older. No advantages were seen for either the adoptive parents or the birthparents. Little empathy for the birthmother was shown in either case, and neither adoptive couple saw themselves as benefiting from knowing the birthmother.

Families with Semi-Open Adoptions

Adoptive parents who had chosen to have a semi-open adoption had generally shared pictures or letters; in only one case had a face-to-face meeting occurred. These families indicated that not knowing the birthmother allowed them to feel more comfortable, protected from the emotional distress of knowing her, and able to develop a positive fantasy about the birthmother. They also suggested that knowledge of the birthmother could be confusing to the child.

These parents felt that traditional adoptions are problematic for the entire triad. Adoptive parents commented that a disadvantage of traditional adoptions is the inability to meet the birthparents causing an increased likelihood of the adopted child searching for his or her birthparents. Similarly, birthparents noted that in traditional adoptions the child will always wonder who his or her birthparents were.

These birth and adoptive parents seemed satisfied with their semi-open adoptions. The adoptive parents were pleased to know that their children's birthmothers were being given updates on the well-being of the children they placed for adoption, and they were happy to have information on the current status of their children's birthmothers. However, one cautious adoptive mother stated, "The less you know, the better." The birthmothers were pleased to have some information about their children and to feel secure that the adoptive parents were happy as well. The difficulties with semi-open adoptions cited by the adoptive parents included fear that the birthmother might want the child back and problems that might occur when much more information is available on one child's birthmother than on a sibling's.

The birthmothers were pleased to have information, but they seemed to want more: "You always want to have a little bit more." "Giving up the child, seeing the picture drives you crazy. You want to see more. It helps to see pictures, but it's hard too." "My only joy is knowing I'll see her some day."

Families with Fully-Disclosed Adoptions

The ten families with fully-disclosed adoptions in the study had shared identifying information and had ongoing personal contact of some type. Adoptive parents who had chosen this option believed that it is in the best interest of the child to have information about the child's birthparents. They believed that "if you know the birthparents, you don't have to fear that they would snatch the children," and "you know what sort of people the birthparents are." Birthparents noted that openness means that they have no fear, no unknowns, and an honest relationship. When a birthmother has nightmares or dreams, she can pick up the phone and see how the child is. "You have a bond with the family through the child." "He'll always be able to relate back to where he's really from — his parents. If he has questions, he'll be able to ask me. It's the perfect solution." At the same time, some birthparents expressed an interest in overseeing the raising of their children.

Although many adoptive parents saw no disadvantages to openness, two primary concerns emerged: the problem with the additional time and effort required to maintain the relationship, and the need to have a mature birthmother. The disadvantages in openness cited by birthparents centered around the continuing pain they experience in seeing their child. "You have a tendency to think: Gee, if I had only kept her." "Getting close and knowing you can't have him—he's not yours." "Sometimes you want the child back more and more, but you just have to discipline yourself."

Most of the adoptive parents in the group chose fully-disclosed openness with ongoing contact because they felt it was in the best interests of the child. Although they did not feel that they were offered the option to have a traditional adoption, they typically started out with a semi-open situation and gradually progressed to fully-disclosed openness as they established a relationship with the birthparent(s). Some adoptive parents were strongly in favor of their situation: "It's the right thing for all adoptive parents." "Birthparents chose openness because they wanted to know how the child was and wanted the child to know them." "I would have kept the child if I couldn't have openness—I can't imagine not knowing where the baby is and how she's doing."

When adoptive parents discussed the perceived impact openness in general has, they noted that both children and birthparents will have ongoing contact with each other and will experience less pain. However, when discussing the impact on their own situations, several reservations were expressed. For example, one mother stated:

> Sometimes I think I'm tired of sharing. It's getting ready for the visits. The kids will fight and punch each other and you say, "Oh Lord, please don't do this in front of them." When they leave, I say, "Whew, that's another visit over with."

Birthparents believed that open adoptions have a positive impact on the children since they will know where they came from and will understand the birthparents' motives for placing them. For themselves, the birthparents noted that the adoptive family became an extended family. One birthparent noted that she planned to use the adoptive mother as a support unit when she had her own children.

Several birthparents expressed fear about having to explain the relinquished child to their later-born children.

In comparing the responses given by families in the three groups, it is striking that each set of parents felt that their type of adoption was the best situation, and each family was very complimentary of the agency's role in their adoption. It is likely that this satisfaction is due to the thoroughness of preparation offered by the agency before adoption. Moreover, cognitive dissonance theory (Festinger, 1957) would predict that even if parents were opposed to the position of the agency on openness, their desire to adopt may be strong enough to overpower any objections. In order to reduce dissonance then, these parents may seek out information that confirms their point of view and become advocates of the degree of openness chosen. Since birthparents often choose the adoptive parents for their child in open situations, cognitive dissonance theory would predict that the birthparents would be satisfied both with the child's adoptive parents and with the type of adoption chosen.

Risks and Benefits of Differing Degrees of Openness

The traditional adoption situation appears to allow the adoptive parents to take full parenting responsibility for their children and to deal as much or as little with adoption issues as they wish. Depending on the parents, this situation might permit adoptive parents to restrict communication with the child about his or her adoptive status and heritage. Some concern is expressed for the child's right to know about his or her birthparents, but the adoptive parents will not likely encourage the child's searching unless the child presses for it. If the adoptive parents are noncommunicative with the child about the adoption, identity issues in adolescence may present challenges for the entire family (McRoy, Grotevant & Zurcher, 1986). In the traditional situation, the birthparent loses all contact with the child and all information about the child. Research evidence suggests that relinquishment is very painful and has a profound psychological impact on the birthmother's self-concept (Fonda, 1984) as it represents a permanent separation initiated by the relinquishing mother

(Rynearson, 1982). Despite myths to the contrary, birthmothers never forget the child they placed for adoption (Silber & Speedlin, 1983; Lindsay, 1986).

Semi-open adoptions appear to provide benefits to all parties in the adoption triad. The adoptive parents are insulted from interference in their lives with the child, but at the same time, they are in contact with the birthparent(s) and facilitate a communication link between birthparent and child. The birthparents in semi-open adoptions benefit by having the information that they appear to want the most: the knowledge that the child is in a loving environment and is happy and healthy. Although the birthparent may desire more information about the child, a more open situation is not necessarily less painful for them. In fact, ongoing contact appeared to be stressful for a number of the birthmothers interviewed in this study. Benefits to the child include the availability of communication with his or her birthparents and knowledge about his or her heritage. Depending on the specific individuals involved, the door may be open for contact between child and birthparents when the child is of legal age.

Fully-disclosed open adoptions involving ongoing contact appear to benefit the children and the birthparents more fully than the adoptive parents. The children have the love and attention of another adult and come to know the birthparent as a real (as opposed to a fantasized) person. The birthparent has access to the child and can watch him or her grow up. This situation evokes mixed emotions in birthparents: it is reassuring to know that the child is happy and well taken care of; however, it is also painful to see your child and know that you cannot have him or her. In some cases, ongoing contact seemed to encourage the birthparent's fantasy that the child might return to live with them. Unlike the birthmothers in the semi-open situations, the birthmothers in the fully-disclosed open adoption group often felt close to their adoptive families and felt as if they were a member of the family. Although the role that they named was as an "aunt" or a "friend," the interviews and observations of the researchers suggested that some of the birthmothers were more like older daughters of their adoptive parents. They sought advice from their child's adoptive parents and often relied on them for emotional support. The benefits to the adoptive parents seem somewhat less clear. The greatest benefit is that it gives them a realistic picture of the birthparent and prevents stereotyping.

LIMITATIONS

The findings of this study strongly suggest that the degree of openness desirable in any particular case is a highly individual matter. No one type of adoption can be regarded as "best" for every family situation. For some families, traditional adoptions may be problematic and for others semi-open or fully-disclosed openness would not be preferable.

It should be noted, however, that the findings of this study are limited by the sample. Only 17 families from one private adoption organization in the state of Texas were interviewed. Observations and conclusions cannot be generalized to all adoption agencies or families. Further study is needed with different agencies in other geographical areas in the effort to better understand the benefits and limitations of openness in adoptions practice.

The sample selection process was also a methodological limitation of the study. Since birthparents had to be first matched with corresponding adoptive parents in order to be included in the study and had to be contacted by letter or phone, only families who had kept in touch with the agency were selected for participation. Families who could easily be reached by the agency were likely to have had a very positive experience with their adoption and were more likely to volunteer to participate in the study. The self-selection process may have tended to bias the results in favor of the families who were pleased with the degree of openness they had selected.

The consequences of openness for adopted children in this study remains unknown, because the children were too young to be interviewed. A longitudinal study of the impact of openness on all members of the triad is highly recommended.

IMPLICATIONS FOR PRACTICE AND POLICY

In spite of the limitations, the findings of this study have implications for adoption policy. Although offering options based on each family's circumstances seems preferable, agencies which choose to offer differing degrees of openness to their adoptive and birthfamily clients must also be aware of the practice implications of such a policy. Both semi-open and fully-disclosed adoptions have a life-long impact on all members of the adoption triad as well as on the adoption agency.

During the adoption preparation process, adoption workers must be able to critically assess what, if any, degree of openness a family can handle. Similarly, birthparents must be screened to determine which form of openness would be most beneficial to them. Since some families are able to handle open adoptions easier than others, it may be necessary to develop very specific assessment tools and procedures to reevaluate their readiness for openness.

In most cases of fully-disclosed adoptions, the decision to reveal identifying information is made solely by birth and adoptive parents. Even in agencies in which identifying information is shared by the adoption agency at the time of adoption, agency personnel are only involved in the initial meetings. As arrangements for later meetings are often made independent of the agency, it is critical that workers prepare and educate their adoptive and birthfamilies prior to the adoption about the advantages and disadvantages of full-disclosure. They must be aware that, as of this date, the impact of ongoing contact on the child is still unknown. Members of adoptive families should be fully informed about the possible problems that may arise and given an opportunity to discuss the future implications of such a decision, should they wish to opt for more or less contact. Individual and group post-adoption counselling services must be offered to both adoptive and birthfamilies to help them cope with the emerging problems which may develop in a situation of a fully-disclosed adoption. Agency administrators must also assess the fiscal considerations of this required postadoption program.

Until there is sufficient longitudinal research data on the impact of ongoing contact on the adopted child, agencies may wish to develop guidelines for open adoptions which are in keeping with the child's cognitive developmental level (e.g., Brodzinsky, Singer & Braff, 1984). Families should be advised as to what kind of contact, if any, they might consider between their adopted child and birthparents, depending on the child's developmental stage.

When offering semi-open adoptions, the agency makes a commitment to serve as intermediary between birth and adoptive parents for life, since information, pictures, gifts, and letters are typically exchanged through the agency. For some workers, this postadoption responsibility is added to their existing preadoptive parent preparation or birthparent counselling. This expanded case load may produce added stress for social workers. In addition, the workers need to be trained to serve as intermediaries should adoptive families wish to increase or decrease the degree of openness in the adoption as the child gets older. Moreover, agency workers must be aware that birthmothers or adoptive parents may feel abandoned if their workers leave the agency, especially in semi-open situations in which the worker has served as the go-between.

Because parents in traditional adoptions typically receive little birthparent information to pass along to their child, agencies should encourage adoptive families to preserve carefully any information given to them in a scrapbook or baby book. Should the need arise for more information, adoptive families must feel free to contact the agency at any time.

The agency must also educate birthparents as to the necessity of placing accurate and complete medical and background information on both birthparents in the child's files. Birthparents must also be offered the option of leaving letters or other kinds of nonidentifying information in the files as well as be informed of any state or national adoption registries whose services they may wish to use in the future.

Any change in adoption agency practice will require time and money and will create extra work for agency personnel. At first, some adoption workers and administrators may find change stressful. However, the resulting benefits to members of the adoption triad—birthparents, adoptive parents and adopted children—will make changes within agencies worthwhile.

REFERENCES

Brinich, P. (1980). Some potential effects of adoption on self and object representations. In A. Solnit, R. Eissler, A. Freud, M. Kris & P. Neubauer, (Eds). *The psychoanalytic study of the child*. New Haven: Yale University Press.

Brodzinsky, D. M., Singer, L. M. & Braff, A. M. (1984). Children's understanding of adoption. *Child Development, 55*, 869-878.

Campbell, L. H. (1979). The birthparent's right to know. *Public Welfare, 37* (3), 22-27.

Children's Home Society of California. (1984). *The changing picture of adoption*. Los Angeles: Author.

Colon, F. (1978). Family ties and child placement. *Family Process, 17*, 189-312.

Cliff, K. (1983). *Adoption law reviews mixed.* San Antonio Express, September 16.

Curtis, P. (1986). The dialectics of open versus closed adoption of infants. *Child Welfare, 65* (5), 437-445.

Festinger, L. (1957). *A theory of cognitive dissonance.* New York: Harper and Row.

Fonda, A. B. (1984). *Birthmothers who search: An exploratory study.* Unpublished doctoral dissertation. California School of Professional Psychology, Berkeley.

Foster, A. (1979). Who has the 'right' to know? *Public Welfare, 37* (3), 34-37.

Harrington, J. D. (1979). Legislative reform moves slowly. *Public Welfare, 37* (3), 49-57.

Kirk, H.D. (1959). A dilemma of adoptive parenthood: Incongruous role obligations. *Marriage and Family Living, 21* (4), 316-328.

Kirk, H.D. (1964). *Shared fate: A theory of adoption and mental health.* New York: Free Press.

Kirk, H.D. (1981). *Adoptive kinship: A modern institution in need of reform.* Toronto: Butterworth Co.

Kraft, A. D., Palombo, J., Mitchell, D. L., Woods, P.K., Schmidt A. W. & Tucker, N.G. (1985). Some theoretical considerations on confidential adoptions, part III. The Adopted Child. *Child and Adolescent Social Work.* Human Sciences Press.

Lindsay, J. W. (1986). *Open adoption: A caring option.* Buena Park, CA: Morning Glory Press.

McRoy, R.G., Grotevant, H.D. & White, K.L. (1985). *Openness in Adoption: Consequences and Issues.* Final Report prepared for Lutheran Social Services of Texas.

McRoy, R.G., Grotevant, H.D. & Zurcher, L.A. (1986). *The development of emotional disturbance in adopted adolescents.* Final Report prepared for the Hogg Foundation for Mental Health.

McRoy, R.G. & Zurcher, L.A. (1983). *Transracial adoptees: The adolescent years.* Springfield, IL: Charles C. Thomas Publishers.

Pannor, R. & Baran, A. (1984). Open adoptions as standard practice. *Child Welfare, 63* (3), 245-250.

Rynearson, E. K. (1982). Relinquishment and its maternal complications: A preliminary study. *American Journal of Psychiatry, 139* (3), 338-340.

Sanders, P. & Sitterly, N. (1981). *Search aftermath and adjustments.* Author.

Silber, K. & Speedlin, P. (1983). *Dear birthmothers: Thank you for your baby.* San Antonio, TX: Corona Publishing Co.

Sorich, C. & Siebert, R. (1982). Toward humanizing adoption. *Child Welfare, 61* (4), 207-216.

Sorosky, A. D., Baran, A. & Pannor, R. (1975). Identity conflicts in adoptees. *American Journal of Orthopsychiatry, 45* (1), 18-27.

Sorosky, A. D., Baran, A. & Pannor, R. (1984). *The adoption triangle.* New York: Anchor Press: Doubleday.

Triseliotis, J.B. (1973). *In search of origins: The experiences of adopted people.* Boston: Routledge and Keegan Paul.

Zeilinger, R. (1979). The need vs. the right to know. *Public Welfare, 37* (3), 44-48.

Placement Disruptions:
Perspectives of Adoptive Parents

Deborah Valentine
Patricia Conway
Jerry Randolph

SUMMARY. As part of a larger study of adoptive families and their adopted children, the authors conducted in-depth, personal interviews with 18 adoptive families who experienced an adoption disruption. In addition to feeling ill-prepared for the adoptive placement, parents indicated that they felt isolated and alienated during the child's placement and deeply traumatized during and following the disruption. Implications for social work practice are suggested.

In recent years, adoption has become an option for an increasing number of children. Prior to the mid 1960s any child over the age of two-years-old could be labeled "hard to place" and school age children and sibling groups were seldom considered adoptable. Children with medical, behavioral, learning or emotional handicaps were also considered unsuitable for adoptive placement (Jones, 1979). This has changed during the last decade. Children may be referred to as having special needs, but are no longer considered unadoptable.

Concern about children experiencing multiple placements, "foster care drift" and unpredictable and unstable living arrangements has given rise to the practice of permanency planning—the process of taking prompt, decisive action to maintain children in their own homes or place them permanently with other families (Maluccio & Fein, 1983).

While disruption rates for infant adoption are under 3%, those for special needs children may be as high as 23%. Evidence of increasing rates of second adoptions also suggest higher disruption rates (Barth et al., 1986). Because the number of children with special needs that are being placed in adoptive homes has increased, concern about the prevention of adoption disruptions has also increased. Persons familiar with the adoption experience are well aware of the emotional, psychological and financial cost of placement disruptions.

In 1985, representatives of three adoption agencies in South Carolina (two public and one private nonprofit) expressed concern about the number of adoption disruptions occurring among children placed in adoptive homes who fall into the special needs category. During the three year period 1982, 1983 and 1984, the three agencies reported a total of 122 disruptions. In collaboration with these adoption agencies and with the financial support of The Duke Foundation, the authors conducted a research project designed to describe characteristics of disrupted adoptive placements. Information was gathered from three sources: case records, interviews with adoption workers, and interviews with adoptive parents who experienced a placement disruption. The results of the research component describing characteristics of disrupted placements from data gathered from case records and through adoption worker interviews are described elsewhere (Valentine, Conway & Randolph, in press). The results of in-depth interviews of adoptive parents who experienced a disrupted adoption placement are described here.

VIEWS ON PLACEMENT DISRUPTIONS

The primary source of information utilized to increase understanding of disrupted adoptive placements has been professionals in the adoption field. Adoption workers, administrators, and other professionals have disseminated descriptions and interpretations of the disruption experience through professional journals and presentations at professional conferences. Furthermore, when research on adoption disruptions are conducted, data from case records are typically utilized. This information is prepared and written by professionals in the adoption field. The "professional" perspective of the etiology and experience of adoption disruptions is widely accepted as accurate and is used to establish agency policy and guide practice. For example, the professional literature identifies several characteristics of adoptive parents and families which contribute to an increased likelihood of an adoption disruption. These include: unresolved infertility issues; unusual motives for adoption such as replacement of a dead child or an expression of "child saving;" parental attitudes such as excessive concern with the child's behavior and birth parents; highly critical, rigid, inflexible and punitive parental styles; inexperience with parenting; parents who are uncommitted to the adoptive placement or the adopted child; and/or a poor or unstable marital relationship (Valentine, Randolph & Conway, in press, Barth et al., 1986).

Furthermore, although needs of adoptive parents are acknowledged, many professionals in the adoption field perceive themselves as primarily an advocate for the child. Professional advocates of the "no-child-is-unadoptable" position, for example, maintain that "some disruptions are inevitable when placing children for adoption . . . the disruption rate is likely to increase as placement of special needs children increases" (Roberts, 1981, p. 2). Donley (1981) states that "disruption is not necessarily a devastating experience. In fact, it can have a positive end result." Presumably, Donley is speaking on behalf of the child and not the adoptive parent. Disruption is viewed as an *interruption* in the process leading to the long-range goal of permanent placement of the child. Following the disruption, the plan for the child is *re-placement* with another adoptive family (Roberts, 1981). Clearly the focus is the child. The loss, pain, and sense of failure experienced by adoptive parents is not emphasized, nor is the obstacle to fulfillment of the long-range goal of "parenting" a child mentioned. Quite the contrary, social workers may underestimate the feelings of loss and failure experienced by adoptive parents who experience a disrupted placement. Festinger (1986) reports in her study of 183 adoptive placements in New York City that caseworkers who were involved in an adoption disruption were "quite disappointed about what happened, and sometimes openly angry at the family. In fact, in two out of three cases, they (caseworkers) stated that they would not place another child for adoption with these families. In contrast, their outlook on the child was quite different, for in most instances, workers need to find another adoptive home for the majority of the children" (p. 40).

The re-placement concept is clearly the intended objective for the child, not for the adoptive parents, even if they desire re-placement. For example, marketing strategies are currently being developed and advocated as a way to attract other families to serve as adoptive parents to these multiple-placed children (Coyne, 1986). The potentially devastating consequences for adoptive parents and families do not appear to be given sufficient consideration.

One may argue the soundness of adoption practice which underestimates the negative consequences of multiple placements for the child; however, this is a debate to be argued elsewhere. Rather, it is the position of the authors that professionals practicing in the adoption field do not completely or objectively represent the feelings, perspectives, or experiences of adoptive parents who are being asked to risk "the inevitability of some disrupted placements" or who have already experienced a disrupted placement. Furthermore, the needs of adoptive parents who suffer the emotional consequences of a disruption may not be adequately met.

This discussion will describe the results of a unique component of a larger research project. Information gathered from in-depth interviews of adoptive parents who experienced a disrupted adoptive placement will be presented. Rarely have attempts been made to interview adoptive parents who have suffered a disruption and these perceptions and experiences are vital in increasing our understanding of disruption.

METHODOLOGY

Sample Description

A letter requesting voluntary participation in a research project designed to collect information concerning adoption disruptions from the adoptive parents' point of view was sent to all families that received a child from a South Carolina adoption placement agency and that experienced a disrupted adoptive placement during 1982,

1983, or 1984. For purposes of this study, adoption disruption was defined as the removal of a child any time between adoptive placement and the child's emancipation (Valentine, Conway & Randolph, in press). Three participating South Carolina agencies addressed and mailed the letter of request to a total of 122 families. Families agreeing to be contacted returned a postcard or personally contacted a member of the research team. Recruitment was conducted in this manner to assure confidentiality.

Eighteen adoptive families agreed to participate in an in-depth personal interview. Three additional parents contacted the research team but decided to withdraw from participation. Reasons for withdrawal included fear that the interview might arouse too much emotional pain, a recent family crisis, and a fear that information from the interview might jeopardize a future adoptive placement. The response rate may have been limited (15%) because the interviews required that a very emotionally sensitive and painful subject be explored and reminders of "failures" be resurrected. Although the 18 families who participated in this study cannot and should not be considered representative of all parents who experienced an adoption disruption, it is extremely important that professionals practicing in the adoption field listen to what these individuals have to say. They describe an experience that has been untold for too long.

Fifteen of the participating families resided in South Carolina. Three families lived out-of-state (North Carolina, Utah, Michigan).

Fourteen of the participating families were two-parent families and four were single-parent families (two single-parent women and two single-parent men). Of the 14 married couples, the average length of marriage was 20 years. The mean age of adoptive mothers was 42-years-old. The mean age of adoptive fathers was 45-years-old. All but one of the adoptive parents had high school degrees, college degrees and/or advanced degrees. Two participating families were black; 16 were Caucasian. Of the 18 participating families, 15 had previously parented or were currently parenting children in their family. Of these 15 families, three had one or more adopted children, 11 had one or more biological children, and one family had both adopted and biological children in the home. Only three participants, all single adoptive parents, had no other children in the home.

A total of 22 children were placed with the 18 participating families: girls were placed with eight families, boys were placed with eight families and sibling groups were placed with two families. A sibling group of four children was placed with one family (ranging in age from 7 to 16-years-old); a sibling group of two teenage children was placed with one family. One family had received an infant. The remaining 15 children ranged in age from 12 to 16-years-old at the time of placement. The average age of the adopted child placed singly was 14.2-years-old. The mean age of all adopted children placed (exclusive of the infant) was 13.8-years-old. Only the infant was physically or mentally handicapped. All of the other children in the adoptive placements were physically healthy. No special medical needs or substantial mental retardation were reported.

In general, the participants who volunteered for the research project were middle aged. If married, the couples had stable, enduring marriages and had parented other children. The majority of the adopted children were physically healthy, intellectually average adolescents.

Participating parents were eager to share their thoughts, perceptions and experiences. They expressed a desire to contribute to the understanding of adoption disruptions. In addition to the wealth of information gathered, the investigators believed that the interviews provided an unintended therapeutic benefit to the participants. Many of the participants expressed gratitude for the opportunity to "ventilate" and "make sense" of the adoption experience. Parents reported that it was helpful to be able to share their experience with someone who was familiar with the adoption process and had time to listen. Only one family reported receiving or being offered any other postdisruption contact or services to assist them in recovering from the loss of their adopted child.

Data Collection

A semi-structured, focused interview schedule was utilized to explore the experience of the participating families. All participation was voluntary and a written consent was obtained. All interviews were conducted by one of two research investigators. Both interviewers have an MSW and a PhD in social work. The interviews lasted from one and one-half to four hours and were conducted during the Summer and Fall of 1985. All but two of the interviews were conducted in the participants' homes or the interviewer's office. Two interviews from families living outside of South Carolina (Utah and Michigan) at the time of the study were conducted on the telephone. The same interview schedule was followed and neither the quantity nor quality of information obtained by telephone appeared to differ substantially from personal interviews.

In both interview conditions, specific questions were asked participants, but latitude was given to interviewers to explore a wide variety of issues and concerns. Participants were asked to describe events and experiences throughout the entire adoption experience: during preplacement preparation, the actual adoptive placement, the time of disruption and the period immediately following the disruption (the interview schedule is available upon request).

The perspectives shared by parents are no more "the truth" or the "complete picture" than are the perspectives of professionals in the adoption field. The experiences portrayed are the perceptions of 18 families.

It is with deep respect that the members of the research team present the experience of the parents and invite the reader to enter their world. The courage and strength of the parents who risked their emotions and shared their time is greatly appreciated.

RESULTS

The description of the results is divided into four sections: preplacement experiences, placement experiences, the disruption experience, and postdisruption experiences. Because the sample is not intended to be representative and the research is highly qualitative, no statistical presentations of the data are appropriate. The results of all interviews were reviewed and general impressions and conclusions in narrative form with statements by participants provided for illustrative purposes are presented.

Preplacement Experience

The preplacement experience includes preplacement preparation of parents and children and the selection and matching of child and adoptive family. Overall, adoptive parents perceived the preplacement preparation classes, home studies, and family interviews as helpful and necessary. The majority of participants felt that nothing more of a general nature could have been done prior to placement that would have better prepared them for the adoptive child or children who were placed in their homes.

When describing the selection of a particular child for their family, however, 11 of the 18 families reported that they were dissatisfied. Although 17 families received a child of the gender they requested, eight of the families received children who were older than originally requested and two families received more children than requested.

> We wanted an 8 to 9-year-old boy. The agency suggested a 10 to 12-year-old. We ended up with a 15-year-old.

Nine families reported receiving a child with behaviors that were specifically identified as unacceptable.

> We specifically said we couldn't handle a sexually active girl. What did we get? A *very* provocative, sexually active 14-year-old girl!

Participants also felt the match between child and family was either poorly made or that characteristics of relative unimportance were given too high a priority.

> They matched on unimportant things. I wanted a child that matched my values and life styles, not my eye color or hair texture or skin shade.

> I think one thing the agency needs to look at is matching backgrounds of family rather than facial features. It is the core of family life, expectations, that matter.

Adoptive parents also speculated that perhaps they were not given accurate or complete information because the caseworker did not know the child.

> We were originally told the oldest was 12, but he was actually 16.

> We saw F. in the newspaper. This was not the same kid we met. He gained four years and 200 pounds in three months. We thought the agency switched kids!

Other parents indicated that they felt they were deliberately misinformed about the extent of the child's emotional and behavioral problems reflected in the following statements.

> We got the impression K. was an all-American boy.

> Worker painted too rosy a picture.

This was further emphasized by participants who suggested that they felt the adoption worker was really in the business of "selling" children. One father commented that he felt that "they were more interested in a placement than a good match." Several parents felt that they were persuaded to accept a child into their home for adoptive placement against their better judgement.

> We were given a sales job.

> We were sold a bill of goods.

> They sold us a child like they'd sell a used car.

> The caseworker gave me a lot of hype.

> . . . false advertisement was used.

> She (the caseworker) talked me into it. I knew I shouldn't. Deep down inside, you know what's wrong or right.

> The worker said, "Just take her home. It will all work out."

The parents reported that they were swept away by the anticipation of becoming parents and responded to the workers' encouragement and to their own desire and eagerness to parent. Children were welcomed into their families despite some hesitancy, however, and reluctance was rationalized.

> We thought maybe we'll give it a try and keep them for awhile.

> The poor things don't have a home, no one wants them and we've got this big house and a lot of love.

Four adoptive families who participated in the study also suggested that the children were ill-prepared for the adoptive placement. Either the children were misinformed about the family or they frankly admitted that they had no desire to be adopted.

> I'm not sure she (adopted daughter) understood what adoption meant.

> He was talked into adoption, but didn't really want a family.

> He was given a sales job. We could have never lived up to what he expected.

> He didn't want to be adopted. He didn't want to change his name and he didn't want people to know anything.

Placement Experience

Despite the stress of acquiring a new family member and possible reluctance to adopt the particular child or children selected for them, 17 out of the 18 adoptive families stated that when the child was placed in their home they began the attachment and bonding process with the adopted child and were committed to adoptive parenting.

> We cared about him. We felt we could bring out the best in him if we gave him a real loving environment.

> We wanted him and we loved him. We loved him like we would a baby from birth.

Early in the placement, some parents experienced several weeks of honeymoon in which the placement went smoothly.

> She was pretty and charming and young and verbal . . . She said first off "I love you, Mommy."

Others experienced surprise or difficulties from the very beginning:

> It was a nightmare from the beginning.

> I knew within 48 hours it wasn't going to work. I needed a preplacement visit and didn't have one.

> We didn't know he smoked until he got here. It didn't occur to me that a kid his age (14-years-old) would be that addicted!

All parents, however, reported that behavioral problems of the adopted child or children eventually emerged. Most felt bombarded with emotional and behavioral difficulties.

> He was defiant, macho and rude — the most unlovable character.

> They sent up a girl that was more of a woman than I knew what to do with.

> She was a 13-year-old going on 25 or 30. Emotionally she was an 8-year-old.

> There was constant uproar. We're not used to this constant upheaval.

> We had been told C. was strong willed, so we expected that. We didn't expect him to take over the house.

As the placement progressed, the behavioral and emotional problems became more evident and the seriousness of the problems intensified. Behaviors of the adopted children as reported by the adoptive parents are listed in Table I.

Even though parents felt prepared to handle many kinds of difficulties and problems, most parents felt inadequate and ill-prepared to parent such extremely disturbed children.

TABLE I

Behaviors of Children in Adoptive Placements Who Later Disrupt

Reported by Adoptive Parents

	N
Sexually Active	9
Very Emotionally Disturbed (animal torture, fire setting, encopresis, hallucinations, murder)	9
Manipulative and Uncooperative (defiance, lying)	9
Poor School Performance and/or Poor School Behavior (failing grades, suspension, expulsion)	8
Explosive Temper, Violent	7
Stealing	7
Inappropriate Sexual Behavior (multiple sexual partners, sexually provocative behavior, sexual assault)	6
Runaway	5
Poor Personal Hygiene (refuse to bathe, wash hair, and/or wear clean clothes)	4
Smokes cigarettes	3
Substance Abuse	1

NOTE: Total equals more than total number of children because more than one behavior was reported for each child.

We were told nothing real specific to help with the tornado down the road.

If they (the agency/worker) had just told me there'd be a storm, I would've brought an umbrella.

Parents simply reported that they were ill-equipped to deal with these *extremely* disruptive behaviors.

How do you parent a child who tortures animals and sets your house on fire? I just didn't know what to do. Do you?

It is a testament to the commitment of these parents to adoptive parenting that they continued to struggle despite the disruptive behaviors of the child and despite the perception of a lack of support from agencies and workers.

I thought this is just a little fella — if I can get through all these hard times (bed-wetting, stealing cars, school failure) we'll have it made.

Toward the end when things were really crumbling around us, he asked, "Why don't you beat me? You don't love me if you don't beat me."

Relationship with Adoption Agency and Worker

Parents did turn to their adoption workers and the agency for support. Sixteen families, however, indicated that the adoption agency or adoption worker was a source of stress during the placement.

The agency was uninvolved, uninformed and unavailable. They don't understand the psychological needs of kids.

We tried to build some kind of bridge but the social worker was very businesslike. She said not to approach this as missionary work . . . that these kids don't appreciate that . . . someone else will take care of them if you don't.

The agency is out of touch with what kids really need. They were only concerned with the insignificant and not the overall well-being of the child.

The worker said, "I don't have time to talk to you."

Social worker only visited twice in nine months saying, "Call if you have a problem." When a crisis arose, she'd show up one week later.

It is not helpful to hear from a professional that this is normal adolescent behavior. Stealing and promiscuity is not normal adolescent behavior.

The worker said, "Once you get a child for adoption, she's yours. I wash my hands — it's your parental responsibility just like a birthchild would be."

We were supposed to have post-placement meetings once a month but we only had three meetings in the entire year.

Six families did report that they found that at least one of their adoption workers was helpful, concerned and/or available.

We had a wonderful worker — very helpful.

Our worker was always there when we needed him. He gave good sound advice.

The length of adoptive placement represented in this study ranged from one month to 33 months. The mean, mode, and median length of placement was 12 months. Six families reported a frenzy of behavioral and emotional difficulties in the months immediately prior to adoption finalization (in most cases at one year). In six cases, disruption occurred during the 11th or 12th month of placement.

Disruption Experiences

In nine families, the parents requested that the child be removed from the home. In nine of the cases, the child requested a new placement or the placement agency or another agency (law enforcement) removed the child.

The decision to disrupt the placement was agonizing for eight of the nine families who made the decision.

> During the Christmas holidays, I prayed daily, all day long. "What can I do?" Then it dawned on me. I'm trying to correct something that can't be corrected. They don't belong here.

> I just couldn't live with all the unhappiness. Some people learn to live that way. I can't stand it.

> We have to give her up because she was making a disaster of our family. There was a riot wherever we went.

> I wish they could have settled down so we could have kept them. I loved them a lot.

> We loved him and had his best interests at heart but couldn't keep him.

In four other families, parents reported that caseworkers responded to the child's request for a change of placement.

> The child was allowed to try on placements like she was trying on clothes.

> B. requested the disruption one month before legalization and (the agency) removed him immediately without the courtesy of explaining the reasons. He left on the day that he called me "dad" for the first time.

In three cases, the child chose not to legalize the adoption.

> We were the fourth family that tried to adopt J. He rejected each of them before finalization and it was no different with us . . . he said over and over again that this adoption won't work and he was right.

> She kept saying, "If Mommy and Daddy can't love me, why should you?" We tried to fill the void in her life, to take the place of her parents, but she wouldn't let us.

> You've got to have commitment and some kids just don't bond.

Two families reported that caseworkers removed children from the adoptive placement without consulting or informing them. One child was picked up from school and the adoptive parents never saw her again. In both families, an adoptive parent was accused by the child of sexually provocative behavior. The families were very angry that they did not have the opportunity to discuss this accusation with either the child or the worker. In both cases, the accusations were never directly addressed. Parents felt that the child manipulated the worker and was allowed to make decisions regarding placement that were beyond their maturity or ability.

Postdisruption Experiences

The months following the disrupted placement were extremely traumatic for 16 of the 18 families represented in this study. Clear evidences of grieving, loss and crisis were apparent.

> I felt like a failure. I felt terrible, very hurt. I missed him. I'm depressed. I hurt when I think that G. doesn't have a home.

> She will be in my heart forever. The disruption was worse than a death because she's not gone. I'll always wonder.

> It's like a death . . . traumatic . . . I need to heal for awhile. I need to rest.

> She's gone but she's not.

> We got sick at heart when he left. I grieved, my wife was relieved.

> The loss is so painful. It is like a death. I will never adopt again. I am so afraid it would happen again.

Sixteen of the families indicated that they would have benefited from some form of postdisruption support. Parents stated that knowledge of the child's well-being and/or counseling specifically designed to help them deal with their own loss would have been appreciated.

> We needed help afterwards. They took such care before and then no care was available after she left.

I wish the adoption agency would develop procedures to un-adopt.

The caseworker told me that she had no time.

The worker said: "The child has been in three placements in three months and is not eating. I hope you're happy."

Other adoptive parents were more hopeful. They felt that their love and kindness contributed to the child's sense of well-being and adoptive placement should not be the only measure of success. Six families felt that the adoption may not have been successful but the relationship was successful. These families reported that they still maintain regular contact with the child. One family allowed the child to get married in their home and two others continue to provide periodic financial support.

IMPLICATIONS FOR SOCIAL WORK PRACTICE

The results of the interviews conducted with adoptive parents who experienced an adoption disruption in South Carolina between 1982-1984 have been presented. Issues and problems mentioned by participants as increasing the likelihood of disruption or increasing stress for the adoptive parents are highlighted. Suggestions for social work practitioners in addressing those problematic areas are presented.

Although the authors do not imply that adoption workers show unconcern or disrespect for adoptive parents, one overriding suggestion emerging from the data is that practitioners could better assist the entire adoptive family by more fully understanding and empathizing with the adoptive parent experience. An increased effort towards "tuning in" would benefit adoptive families throughout the adoption process. Workers who listen carefully and believe parents' preferences for a particular age child, or a nonsexually active child, for example, convey respect for the prospective parent's ability to assess the capabilities and limitations of their family. Persuasive, high powered marketing techniques may increase the number of adoptive placements; however, it may also increase the number of placement disruptions.

Workers who trust and empathize with adoptive parents also benefit the adoptive child. Living with a child for 24 hours per day provides families with a perspective of the child that is not available to a social worker or the child's therapist. This information can be extremely valuable as treatment plans are being designed to meet the needs of the child. Adoption workers who listen carefully to parents' description of their adoptive child's behavior can reduce stress in several ways. Parents appreciate adoption workers who listen carefully and are empathic, respectful and nurturing. Hearing that the behavior of the child is "normal adolescent behavior" is not helpful. This implies that parents cannot distinguish normal from extreme behavior. It also implies that their parenting skills are inadequate if they are unable to manage the child. Workers who acknowledge that most people do not have the skills to parent children with extreme behavioral disorders are in a better position to provide families with the special assistance families need. Strategies for assisting adoptive families might include consultation with experts in behavior management or child psychopathology. Therapists specially trained to treat children dealing with issues of loss, multiple placements, and adoptions might be recommended. Family therapy, marriage counseling, and/or individual therapy for adoptive families can be considered and recommended when appropriate. The awareness that the adoption worker realizes the enormity and stress of parenting a difficult child is supportive to parents. Being able to offer and provide assistance is welcomed.

Family advocacy rather than child advocacy may also be a more appropriate role for social workers in adoption practice. Parents who feel they have the support, understanding and trust of their worker may be able to expend more energy and effort toward making the placement successful than parents who feel misunderstood or unappreciated. Adoptive children who witness consistent, cooperating adults may respond positively. A family advocate may also be in a better position to consider the consequences of a stressful adoptive placement on the entire family as well as the child. The family advocate might consider disrupting an adoptive placement based on the needs of the family as well as on behalf of the adopted youngster, for example.

Current adoption practice which maintains that every child is a suitable candidate for adoption demands reevaluation. Some children's behavior is so destructive or ill-suited for the intensity of family living that a disrupted placement is virtually inevitable. Adoptive families, children and agencies all lose. Adoptive families lose the hope of parenting, children suffer the pain of an additional placement failure and adoption agencies lose families who may have been excellent adoptive parents for a more appropriate child. Adoption workers also report experiencing a sense of failure and loss when a placement disrupts.

Social workers who have the time and flexibility to be available throughout the entire adoptive placement process are appreciated by parents. Visits should be made as promised and support groups should always be available on a regularly scheduled basis despite seasonal or occasional underutilization. Parents should feel secure in the knowledge that support is available during their times of crises, not only at agency or worker convenience. Social work services should also be available during the placement disruption. A worker's empathic acknowledgement of the difficulties and the struggles of adoptive families is healing for both parent and child. It is also important that adoption workers do not underestimate the impact of a disrupted placement on the parents. The disruption may or may not be a tragedy for the child but is most likely experienced as such for the parents.

When a child requests disruption, social workers are in an opportune position to help family members and adopted children process the experience. It is important that each person understand the reasons and perspectives of the other members as much as possible. Recognizing that the time immediately prior to legalization is a particularly vulnerable time for placement disruption, for example. Adoption workers who facilitate family conferences may be in a position to prevent disrupted placements, especially those disruptions requested by the adoptive child.

As a general rule, an adoptive child should never be removed from an adoptive home without discussing the decision with the adoptive parents and the child. Even in uncomfortable situations such as when a child accuses a parent of sexual misconduct, conferences can be beneficial. Parents are entitled to complete and accurate information and an opportunity to respond. Children, especially adolescents, can also benefit from an understanding of problem-solving, consequences and open, honest interchange. In this capacity, social workers can facilitate planful termination procedures when necessary.

Parents request that postdisruption supports be routinely available to all family members who experience a disrupted adoptive placement. If adoption disruptions are to be accepted as one of the inevitable risks of placing children with special needs, the field of adoption practice should take responsibility for providing care and treatment for the children and families who experience the disruption. Post-disruption intervention might include individual or family therapy, support groups, or continued follow-up casework services provided by the adoption worker. Advanced, specialized professional skills are required to provide the suggested services to special needs children and adoptive families. Familiarity and expertise in child development, behavior management, family assessment, and grief and loss are necessary for adoption workers. Direct practice skills in individual, group and family treatment are also essential. Agency support for maintaining the highest professional standards for adoption workers is crucial.

It is important to remember that adoptive parents are ordinary people who have taken on an extraordinary job—the job of caring for special children. The importance of showing respect and utilizing professional skills for both children and parents cannot be overemphasized. One adoptive parent made a plea to all adoption workers:

> Just believe the parents. Don't keep looking for perfect parents. They don't exist.

REFERENCES

Barth, R., Berry, M., Carson, M.L., Goodfield, R. & Feinberg, B. (1986). Contributions to disruptions and dissolutions of older-child adoptions. *Child Welfare. 64*(4), 359-371.
Coyne, A. (1986). Recruiting foster and adoptive families: A marketing strategy. *Children Today. 15*(5), 30-33.

Donley, K.S. (1981). Observations in disruption. *Adoption Disruptions*. (Publication No. 81-30319). Washington, DC.: U.S. Department of Health and Human Services-Children's Bureau.

Festinger, T. (1986). *Necessary risk: A study of adoptions and disrupted adoptive placements*. Washington, DC: Child Welfare League of America.

Jones, M.L. (1979). Preparing the school-age child for adoption. *Child Welfare. 58*, 27-34.

Maluccio, A.N. & Fein E. (1983). Permancy planning: A redefinition. *Child Welfare. 62*, 195-201.

Roberts, B. (1981). *Adoption disruptions*. (Publication No. 81-30319). Washington, DC: U.S. Department of Health and Human Services-Children's Bureau.

Valentine, D., Randolph, J. & Conway, P. (in press). Review of the literature on adoption disruptions: An ecological perspective. *Pediatric Social Work*.

Valentine, D., Conway, P. & Randolph, J. (in press). Adoption disruption: A case record review. *Parenting Studies*.

Post-Legal Adoption Services: A Lifelong Commitment

Marietta E. Spencer

SUMMARY. This article offers a description of the varied functions which well-directed post-legal adoption services can provide for all members of the adoption triad. Adoptive parents, adopted children or adults, and birthparents experience life-long issues and concerns peripheral to the adoption arrangement. These can be positively addressed and alleviated through knowledgeable and timely intervention, through support and problem-solving expertise. Adoptive families are currently built in many ways. It has become widely accepted that informed post-legal adoption services are a must for all child welfare agencies involved with adoption.

Human service professionals are becoming aware of the need for the adoption triad to cope with adoption realities over its lifetime. The demand for attention to this matter comes from all triad participants: adopted adults, adoptive parents, and birthparents, as well as from professionals involved in adoption services. An increased sensitivity to the way the adoption experience touches the lives of all triad members occurred during the 1960s and 1970s. Subsequently, the practices connected with adoption preparation and selection and the brief social services following the placement of children into their new families were critically evaluated. When legalization of the social contract making a child a son or daughter through adoption occurred, professionals considered their task complete. Were they right that no further service attention was in order? Did they indeed understand how families fared, what they felt, experienced, thought, and how they coped? Did adoption professionals know enough about the lifelong implications of adoption to prepare them for it?

TRIAD FOCUSED SERVICES

The need for triad focused services has become increasingly apparent. By listening to clients, learning from them and following-up on provided services, one becomes aware of the need for an expanded, comprehensive, and creative approach to post-legal adoption services. This can be accomplished in numerous ways.

1. *Keeping abreast of social change* applies to the adoption scene. Parents of an 18-year-old adopted in infancy have read the current newspaper and magazine stories, have listened to the media, and are baffled and distraught to hear about "searchers," i.e., adopted adults meeting with birthparents. "Will our child be wanting to do that?" they ask themselves. "We have not been prepared for such an eventuality!" "Are we successful parents because our son and daughter have not asked us any questions about their adoption?" They conclude: "We really do not know what is normal for kids to want to know. Is there a source of information to help us with an answer?" They called their adoption agency and were invited to a workshop designed to bring people up-to-date on present day thinking, changing practices, and controversial viewpoints. A workshop designed to provide counseling and information will enhance participants' skills in listening and communicating and facilitate a better understanding of their own conclusions and feelings.

2. *The sharing of genetic background information* can be a salutary experience. Twelve-year-old Paul asks mother, "How tall do you think I will grow?" and mother replies "I don't know, dear, because you were adopted." When mother and father later talk over this conversation, they begin to chuckle. "We don't know how tall the people in our child's genetic ancestry were — not because we adopted our child, but because our agency did not share with us such information as we now learn we need in parenting." Children, adopted or not, predictably ask questions based on factors of heredity. In modern times, developmental as well as medical and genetic information is helpful to parents and children (Wisconsin Clinical Genetics Center, 1984). Predictive and preventive value of such caringly and accurately collected data are of undisputable value to parents and to the family's community support system.

This family contacted the agency who arranged their child's adoption and found to their pleasure, that they were invited to a background sharing interview. During this session, they not only received well-collected social and medical information on their child's birthparents, but also on the families of both the birthmother and the birthfather. Their child had come along to this interview and wanted very much to understand the reason why adoption had been decided upon for him? What was the reason for the transfer of parental rights? On the way home, he also asked his parents how their decision had been made by them to adopt him? How did they know he was "the right one?" Receiving answers to their questions keeps children from fantasizing and feeling uncertainty (Brodzinski et al., 1981).

Ideally, children should have been helped to integrate their genetic background information in an honest and constructive manner before reaching the age of 14. However, when this does not occur, it is vital that parents create opportunities to share information whenever possible. Such conversations help to make the children feel that they belong and tie the children into the family. Paul's parents were able to meet their son's normal need to understand his genetic background; they also felt better equipped as parents and closer to him.

3. *Intermediary services* which offer adult adoption triad members an opportunity to obtain and exchange updated nonidentifying information from each other by professionals trained and empowered to provide such services are becoming more important.

Lori is seven-years-old. A thorough physical examination shows that she exhibits signs of hypoglycemia and hyperactivity. It would be helpful to understand more about the sugar metabolism in her genetic ancestry and also, some more about behavior patterns there. Her doctor is requesting whatever can be found out from the child's genetic ancestry.

Susan, a birthmother now married, gave birth to a second child. This child shows a birth defect which can be transmissable to the adopted child's children. The adoptive family is apprised of the condition documented by the birthmother's physician and adds the information to the initial background history received when the child joined their family. They will have Ann tested to see whether she is a carrier of the genetic defect, letting the birthmother know the outcome of the tests. Meanwhile, the family has requested the agency to thank the birthmother for having them notified and want her to know that Ann is a chubby, somewhat shy but happy and loved 11-year-old. When tests results came back positive, the agency drew in the state geneticist, who provided expert genetic counseling. Ann's adoptive family also availed themselves of some post-adoption workshops focusing on how and when to deal with adopted children's questions about their genetic ancestry and about how to explain adoption to others.

4. *Outreach* is a recently coined term used in lieu of the old word "searches." Social service agencies frequently keep on file the original and changing addresses of all of their clients, birthparents as well as those of adoptive families. Clients are urged to keep their addresses current with the agency, and to be aware that updated medical and other information concerning them may be of value to the other triad members. Special informational *update* forms were constructed with an input from geneticists, social workers and adoption triad members. Widely used within Minnesota, these forms have also found their way into many other states and even been exported abroad.

Instead of the old concept of "making a search for. . . . " one should now use more constructively "reaching out," "locating" or "seeking to make contact" with birthparents or with the adoptive family so as to obtain information from them or to ask them for an update. When actual letter exchange or face-to-face meetings are requested, however, not all parties agree to enter into such an agreement. It is vital to be represented by a confidential, well-based professional, an experienced impartial go-between, a counselor who serves clients within the law. Each adult party should have the right to waive or protect their own confidentiality.

An adopted person, Eric, 35-years-old, is requesting that an outreach be made for his birthmother. He comes in for an interview, spending two hours drawing upon the experience of the outreach social worker, sharing his thinking and feelings regarding possible outcomes and expectations. Well-collected background information had been shared with Eric by his parents during his growing-up years. Not yet married, he wondered what future children might be like. A meeting with his birthmother and possibly his birthfather would be in order, he thought. His adoptive parents stood by, supportive and willing also to get to know their son's birthkin provided they were agreeable to a meeting. Eric was appreciative for the chance to discuss and weigh the implications for all parties involved. As he laughingly said, "You can't look in Emily Post's book for answers to practical questions such as what to call my birthmother when I meet her!" Eric also wanted to make an informed decision about personal contact with his birthmother. Biographical statements written by adopted persons and birthparents desiring contact with each other help in making a decision regarding going ahead with it or not.

To his surprise, Eric learned from the biographical sketch he received that his birthparents had married after his birth and subsequently had nine more children. But never did they forget that he was their first born, and every family portrait had — unbeknownst to their other nine children — a space left in it for him. When they learned of his request to meet with them, they were overjoyed and acceded to his wish. Meeting Eric filled a void in their lives. Through preparation before the meeting, Eric's birthparents became aware that he would never "rejoin" their own family unit as a 10th child, but is wholly tied in with his parents and the family who adopted him 35 years ago. It takes careful thought to show acceptance and caring in the right way, when adoption triad members connect and grope for achieving comfortable relationships. Contact, follow-up, support, discussion groups resolving issues, and preventing problems have proven useful to all triad members.

Open-ended support group meetings on a monthly basis have also been helpful to birthparents and adopted persons, as well as to parents of adopted individuals. The groups provide the opportunity to sort out expectations from realities, to talk about relationship development, nonrelationships, consequences of the public image, and identity concerns.

Services will be occasionally requested for counseling and sometimes for go-between purposes at various times after triad parties have established contact. Clients may need support to connect with or to disconnect from one another. A successful outcome achieves problem resolution and normalization. Feelings of victimization and "differentness" should be worked through, where such feelings may have been present. The specific question of "Why am I who I am?" should be answered as part of the identity quest of the adopted person. Birthparents must face what was — the birth and the nonparenting decision, however it was made. They may only become fully aware of a great sense of loss over the missed years of parenting upon meeting the grown adopted adult — the birthchild remembered as an infant or as a very young child.

As Evelyn, a birthmother, stated in a support group meeting: "It is so easy for me to idealize what raising Tom might have been like. Fantasy allows me to forget how young I was then and that I had no work skills nor a 'nest' for my baby to bring him home to. Trying to parent him would not have worked out well." An adoptive mother and father, in one of the support group meetings, told of the initial bewilderment they felt when their daughter Sandy voiced an interest in knowing more about her genetic ancestry. Post-legal adoption counseling led them to see their daughter's desire through her eyes. Why should Sandy not have information on her birthkin? When Sandy later wanted to consider a possible meeting with her birthmother, they, as Sandy's parents, thoroughly understood and backed her decision to request an outreach. Preparation and the ability to make an informed decision before taking the step of personal contact is an important contribution post-legal adoption service makes to adoptive families.

5. *Individual and family problem-solving counseling* is a necessary part of post-legal adoption services. Adoption triad members may need to sort out what, if any part, the fact of adoption plays in their concerns. Concerns range from a sense of uncertainty in parenting their adoptive child, to stress in relationships because of a "hidden secret," or of insecurity about whether adoption is an authentic family tie. Outside influences may be unsupportive to the family by adoption, seeing the child not as the "real" child, or not as "their own." By the same token, children may hear from friends that their adoptive parents are not their "real" parents. Words used in connection with adoption are frequently unintentionally negative (Spencer, 1979).

Parents may tell their adopted child that "your mother loved you so much, she gave you up." A playmate might say to the same child: "Your real mother didn't want you, she put you up for adoption." Another child asks the teacher: "Why do you think I was adopted out by my real mother? My mom at home, says she could not take care of me . . . I wonder what was wrong with her that she couldn't? Mom says she doesn't know why. Maybe she was a bad lady . . . or she thought that I was an ugly baby . . . " The words "surrendering a child" or "relinquishing a child" are also experienced negatively by the adoption triad, the child, the birthparent, and the adoptive parent. There is more to adoption than untying a parenting knot. Birthparents and society focus on adoption which reties a knot, by giving parental rights and obligations to new parents who feel ready and able to take on the challenge of raising the child and offer permanent family membership.

Developing a poor sense of identity can result from not being given a sense of clear belonging. Children may suffer confusion about their ancestry and wonder what it may be like. They may explore likeness to themselves or be helped to differentiate themselves from their ancestry. An adopted child should always be tied into his or her family by adoption at all logical points, without dwelling on the adoption fact specifically. Parents might say, "Even if you don't look like me, we sure think alike." Or: "It is wonderful to have a daughter! There is much mother and daughter can do for one another, aside from having a daughter try to borrow mother's sweaters and blouses! I would like to ask your opinion on how we can plan a little vacation just for ourselves, while dad is on his business trip."

6. *The meaning of functional family relationships* should be explained and illustrated as a part of everyday living. Where fitting, genetic heredity should be an open subject, also. Genetics, as a field of study, describes how genes can influence personal health and physical appearance, how genes predispose people to behavioral tendencies, and direct preventive health care. Much has been learned about genetics and genetic counseling in the past few decades. Several studies have looked at populations who are members of the adoption triad and support what workers in the adoption service field have concluded: Genetics is a reality component which, traditionally in our country has been assiduously overlooked. We have given parents with adopted children the wrong prescription for

parenting, by leading them to believe that "all children really need is love and a sense of security" and they will turn out the way the parents want.

It becomes obvious when one begins to comprehend the implications of the genetic component, that well-collected background information on the child's antecedents and on other children born to the birthparents, if indeed there are any, will become a vital help in parenting a child. Adoption workers and pregnancy counseling staffs must understand how and why to collect medical and social genetic ancestry information from the birthmother and birthfather wherever possible. How this information is then written up and presented so as to be usable and useful to adoptive parents is the next step. Their ability to make appropriate use of the facts presented, may well require some preparation in workshops for parents at various stages of their child's development.

7. *Providing transracial and transcultural adoptive families* with knowledge and understanding of the culture or ethnic group from which the child came, should include information about geography, shared physical characteristics, and political issues tied to the international and local scene related to a specific ethnic group — be they Asian, Black, East Indian or of other origin. Custom, values, and history of the respective group from which a child stems, are important for the entire adoptivefamily to learn about (McRoy & Zurcher, 1983; Han & Spencer, 1984).

8. *Coping as a family of mixed ethnic composition* is vital. Rather than singling out a child as "the different one," or sending the child alone to learn about his or her culture or origins, or negating the child's "difference" entirely so as not to have to cope with it all, the entire family should assume an identity as ethnically diverse. Communication skills need to be developed around community relationships and interpersonal dealings. Public relations challenges can be among the most taxing tasks experienced by both parents and children. Extended family members may need to learn how to respond to friends and neighbors who are curious about how their grandchild or cousin became part of the family given differences in appearance or language. Many American grandmothers have pulled out their grandchild's picture, only to see surprise on their friend's faces when they gazed upon the photograph of their Vietnamese or East Indian grandchild. In learning and discussion groups, commu-

nication skills and styles can be explored and selected to match both personality and purpose.

Sometimes children rise to the occasion in creative and ingenious ways, as did a four-year-old girl shopping with her mother at the grocery store.

This child of Latin American descent, dark complected and with shiny black hair, walked next to her blond mother and fair haired brother who sat in the grocery cart. After staring at them while in the check-out line, a curious lady pointed at the baby boy in the cart and turning to the four-year-old Tina, asked: "And who is this?" "This is my brother," answered Tina. The lady contemplated the situation some more and then asked Tina, while totally ignoring the mother. . . . "And what does the father look like?" "Like a frog." Tina was quick to respond. The lady was perplexed — mother was amused. When she recounted the story, she added: "If I had trained Tina to say this, it would have never come out right!" However, there are more serious occasions for which preparation may be in order on how to orient friends, teachers, medical professionals or the public.

9. *Helping children to understand why adoption was planned* for them, what their birthparents were like and sharing details about genetic ancestry may be more of a problem with intercountry adoptions because less well-collected details are likely to be available. Also, adoptive parent's comprehension of the decision-making process and emotional consequences of the adoption decision that took place in a distant land may be more elusive for American parents. Thus, they may be less able to speak to their child authoritatively, with empathy and comfort about these topics. For example, parents who have adopted children from overseas seem to have more difficulty talking about the birthfather of their child than about the birthmother.

10. *Identity and adjustment issues for the transculturally and the transracially adopted child* are complex. Sometimes the adoption factor is neglected, because the more obvious ethnic origin differential takes precedent in facing daily life situations (Feigelman & Silverman, 1983).

Adjustment issues such as social and peer group acceptance of the child, possible health problems and understanding the child's early history of liabilities which predate the adoptive placement are important to consider throughout the adoptive placement. Any and all of these factors will affect the adjustment of the child in the family and community and are important to be addressed as best as possible. Not all of the adjustment problems can be totally over-come and differences in relationship content and quality may have to be accepted, both by the child and by the family. Counseling and support groups may ease stress, encourage more positive coping and provide guidelines for expectations. Positive role models form the same ethnic group can serve to enhance the child's self-image and also offer parents insights into the culture of origin of their son or daughter.

11. *A greater demand for openness* in adoption practice has come about as a result of many changing factors in our society. Over the past few years adoption placement practice has explored innovative ways of providing clients with optional avenues through which to fill their need for information about one another. Parties involved, with all adults consenting can elect either nonidentifying or fully-disclosed information to be shared. The options may involve updating case file information regularly versus face-to-face meetings.

Some of the face-to-face meetings of birthparents and adoptive parents or adopted adults with birthparents take place without sharing names and addresses of the participants. These are called semi-open contacts. Others, where identifying facts are shared, are referred to as fully-disclosed meetings. It is likely that resulting complexities in feelings and in relationships will require ongoing social service availability.

12. *Participants in private or independently arranged adoptions*, as well as relative adoption, frequently do not receive counseling preparation prior to the legal adoption. Availability of such help to triad members at later points should also be offered through post-legal adoption services.

POST-ADOPTION SERVICE CENTER: A MODEL

Practice experience and research efforts suggest that a triad focused approach to adoption services is crucial to a successful adoption process. The development of a comprehensive *Post-Adoption Service Center* is one way to meet the needs of all participants. The service should be comprehensive; that is, it should be triad focused, showing an understanding of both the import of adoption family membership status, loyalties and obligations, and a willingness to deal with the reality and implications of genetic descent. Such comprehensive service centers should address the long-term needs of all children who were adopted with equal emphasis. In that way, American infant adoptions, the adoption of older children, sibling groups, or other children for whom it was more difficult to find families, children adopted from other countries would be deemed equally deserving of specialized services, problem solving along the way of growing up, and eligibility for financial subsidies when necessary. Their adoption would thus fulfill the very promise for permanence that the adoption process initially held out for adoptive families and birthparents.

There are many advantages of the Post-Adoption Center model of providing services over the life cycle of the adoptive family. The number of service cases would allow clients to receive well-rounded and experienced services. Many agencies do not have service volume nor the well-trained post-legal adoption staff to deliver quality services in all areas requiring help. The proposed Center would focus on a wide variety of client concerns, develop special focus support groups, workshops, problem solving sessions, counseling, and crisis intervention.

Practice models and innovative ideas could be developed, tested, and instituted. An exchange of ideas and service styles could be made possible through professional cooperation.

Data collection, case examples, descriptive materials allowing for the analysis of patterns, and dynamics of socio/cultural and behavioral/emotional factors would be recognized and utilized in developing individual and family counseling interventions. Results of post-legal adoption services research would provide direction for pregnancy counseling and the preadoptive counseling of adoptive parents, placement practice, and parent-child selection.

Prevention and problem solving services could also be made available through a Post-Adoption Services Center. These services would be designed to reduce family dysfunction and the number of adoption disruptions. Families who adopt children who enter the social service system via foster care, treatment facilities, or through the courts are at increased risk for family breakdown. Children who suffer physical abuse or sexual molestation are also more difficult to parent. Peer group pressure pose a problem for all children; adoption lends additional complexity to the already difficult modern child rearing situation.

Service to clients with special needs could also be addressed by the proposed Center. Clients in remote areas of the state, for example, could receive consultative and training assistance from a knowledgeable central Post-Adoption Center. Special meetings with client special interest groups could also be held.

A Post-Adoption Services Center should also provide resources and impetus for the establishment of a State-wide Post-Legal Adoption Council. Such Councils could be formed among local resource persons from other professional settings who may share their experiences in working with adoption triad members. Included, for example, may be professionals from school settings, churches, scout troops, summer camps, and various treatment facilities. Such Post-Legal Adoption Councils might become a body which would develop a speakers' bureau, work on educational materials, and on community organizations such as the National Committee for Adoption, the Child Welfare League, and the National Council on Family Relations and could be provided by a Post-Adoption Center.

SUMMARY

Parenting problems frequently are exacerbated by any or all of the complex components described earlier causing insecurity, a sense of dislocation, and a diminished sense of ability to cope with the child and with the public's view of their child and the family unit. These are not psychiatric problems, nor are they caused by social pathology. They are problems that can be helped by better informed adoption perspectives, community organization, public education, and advocacy focusing on normalization of adoption in our society. The financial base for such services can come from multiple sources.

It is apparent that post-legal adoption services cover a significant variety of potential areas of concern. These services should be designed to enhance family adaptation and adjustment, domains where the essential elements of post-adaption issues lie. These are to be seen as problems not for the adopted person alone, but for the entire triad membership. It is clear that adoption does not represent social pathology but is rather a socially accepted, legally supported family-building method involving a life-long commitment. As in other human situations, some of the individuals who are members of the triad may have personal and/or relationship issues complicated by adoption. The social work professional challenge is to help clarify and normalize adoption triad client concerns.

REFERENCES

Brodzinski, D., Pappas, C., Singer, L. & Braff, A. (1981). *Journal of Pediatric Psychology, 6*(2), 177-189.

Feigelman, W. & Silverman, A. (1983). *Chosen children: New patterns of adoptive relationships*. New York: Praeger Press.

Han, Hyun-Sook & Spence, M. (1984). *Understanding my child's Korean origins*. St. Paul: Children's Home Society of Minnesota.

McRoy, R. & Zurcher, L. (1983). *Transracial and inracial adoptees: The adolescent years*. Springfield, IL: C. Thomas.

Spencer, M. (1979). The terminology of adoption. *Child Welfare. 57*, 451-459.

Wisconsin Clinical Genetics Center (1984). *Genetic family history: An aid to better health in adoptive children*. Madison, WI.

Teleconference Technology in Adoption: Utilizing Educational Television in Adoption Preparation

Robert L. Howell

SUMMARY. Through the use of an innovative curriculum and tele-conference technology, the Children's Bureau of South Carolina has joined forces with South Carolina Educational Television to make adoption preparation classes readily accessible to clients throughout the state. Teleconferencing originates from a centrally located studio and participants attend at designated technical education sites throughout the state. The curriculum is consistent with the higher education model of obtaining basic or core education before progressing to specialized training. This article describes the curriculum and the use of closed circuit interactive teleconferencing for individuals and couples who are attending classes pertaining to core information basic to all adoptions.

The Children's Bureau of South Carolina (the Bureau) was chartered as a private adoption agency in 1909. It became a separate state agency in 1930 mandated by law to design and implement statewide comprehensive adoption services for children and families in South Carolina. In its continuing effort to provide efficient and effective adoption services for the citizens of South Carolina, the Bureau has developed a unique preparation process called CORE and TRACK. The development and implementation of the CORE and TRACK curriculum enables the agency to utilize South Carolina Educational Television network in its effort to bring preparation workshops to local communities through closed circuit tele-conference facilities located throughout the state.

CORE AND TRACK

Since it reflects the times and the culture of which it is a part, adoption practice has been in an endless process of change. For example, in ancient Babylon, adoption law enabled a family to acquire a son to continue the family lineage, learn the trade of the adoptive father and perform religious rites for the adopter after his death (Benet, 1976). Since providing a male heir was not a major consideration during the Middle Ages in Europe, adoption was almost nonexistent. Instead, the feudal lord protected and supported his vassals who, in turn, supplied the needed labor (Brooks & Brooks, 1939).

Prior to the 20th century, officials believed that permitting adoption would condone and encourage a parent's abandonment of his or her children. The first adoption law in England was not passed until 1926. In the early years of the United States, children were seen as a source of labor. Child placement was designed to benefit adults rather than children (Brooks & Brooks, 1939). Since the early laws of the United States were modeled after the laws of England, it wasn't until the years from 1850-1950 that the beginnings of an interest in the care and protection of orphaned children in the United States was evident (Fink, 1949). In 1920 the nationwide child advocacy organization, the Child Welfare League of America, was founded and from that point on, the main purpose of agency adoption has been to care for the best interest of the child (Brooks & Brooks, 1939).

Individual, investigatively-oriented home studies of prospective adoptive couples were typical in the early years of adoption practice. It is only a recent commitment to the importance of a permanent home for all children which contributes to the current emphasis on placing children who have not traditionally been considered adoptable in adoptive homes. The Bureau responded to this commitment by developing an educational or workshop format for prospective adoptive parents. The family preparation workshop emerged as an effective and useful method for preparing applicants for adoptive parenthood. As the family preparation workshops evolved, alternate techniques were explored and a two-part group educational preparation process emerged called CORE and TRACK preparation.

CORE WORKSHOPS

The first series of educational sessions contains information that is common to all adoptive placements (infant, older child, child with disabilities, sibling groups, international and so forth). This series of workshops is referred to as CORE material and is presented in a group format. Approximately eight families are selected to participate and attend a CORE Workshop series. CORE material provides basic knowledge about adoption that is essential before an applicant can make a commitment to become an adoptive parent.

Intended as beginning preparation for adoption, the CORE Workshops of the family study process assist the family in anticipating the needs of an adopted child and the differences inherent in adoptive parenthood. The process fosters growth and change in attitudes and expectations through increased understanding of what is involved in adoption and the characteristics of the children available for adoption. Group participants define their own strengths and weaknesses, become aware of their own flexibility, their capacity to grow and develop as adoptive parents, and their readiness for adoption at this point in time. Applicants who have completed the agency's preliminary investigative requirements, basic information questionnaire, medical and financial reports, references, and an arrest and child abuse or neglect history check and are considered by their social worker to be candidates for preparation for adoption participate in the CORE Workshop. The social worker and the applicants clarify, in writing, the purpose, expectations, structure and format of the CORE Workshop. Individual family preparation is an option only available to applicants by special permission because of unusual circumstances. It is clear to applicants that the group preparation will be followed by individualized follow-up.

The CORE Workshop is closed to new members after the first session has begun. It consists of four sessions scheduled once per week. Each session lasts approximately two hours. The following topics are covered at each session.

Session 1. The first session introduces material pertaining to the laws, policies and procedures of the adoption process. Criteria for denial of approval, how children are referred to the agency, open adoptions, and legal risks are also presented. A presentation of the characteristics of children currently available for adoption is made. In addition, the needs, concerns, and characteristics of birth parents are described.

Session 2. The second session continues to raise issues pertaining to birth parent services. The film "I'm 17 and Pregnant" is shown. A discussion of adoption from the adoptive family's point of view is conducted by social workers. A panel of adoptive parents attend the last part of the session to address issues pertaining to "infertility resolution and adoption."

Session 3. The third session begins with a discussion led by an agency social worker on adoption from the child's point of view. This is followed by a panel consisting of birth parents, adoptive parents and adoptees. The panel discusses the adoption experience as experienced by each component of the adoption triad thus providing a complete picture of adoption.

Session 4. The nature of the changing family is presented in session four. A parenting profile is utilized to help clients evaluate their needs, desires, and capabilities. Decisions regarding the type of child that best matches their family is formulated by exploring preferences and values. A presentation of "The Grafted Tree" by an adoptive mother is presented and a discussion of the influences of heredity and environment on human growth, development, and behavior is conducted.

Following the successful completion of the CORE Workshops, applicants evaluate the CORE Workshops and select the TRACK Workshops that will best help them to complete their adoption preparation.

TRACK WORKSHOP

The second series of interactive workshops led by the client's social worker consists of knowledge, information, and discussion pertaining to specialized adoptive parenting. Applicants may select workshops which focus on adoption of the healthy infant, the older, special needs child and sibling groups, or the child from another country. More than one TRACK Workshop may be attended. A brief description of each TRACK Workshop follows.

TRACK Preparation: Adopting the Healthy Infant or Toddler

The purpose of this one session preparation workshop is to familiarize prospective adoptive applicants with the critical issues involved in parenting a healthy infant or toddler. Upon completion of this session, group participants should be familiar with the major roles and responsibilities of parenting, be able to recognize how a child may change their family and life style and be able to recognize their ability to adapt to change and stress.

Specific issues and concerns pertaining to parenting an adopted child includes telling the child about being adopted and the circumstances surrounding the adoption. A discussion of the Bureau's placement process and the role of foster parents in the child's life is also included. A foster parent describes the placement process and is available for questions. Bonding, attachment and separation issues and their importance in the placement procedure and later in their child's growth and development is discussed. This TRACK is adaptable to either individual or group method for applicants with or without other children.

International TRACK

After completing the series of CORE Workshops, individuals and couples desiring to adopt a child from another country participate in the International TRACK. If the family is adopting a relative or child of the same culture or race of one or both of the parents, the social worker facilitates the adoptive home assessment process which includes linkage with U.S. Immigration and Naturalization, brokering necessary translations, and monitoring the process.

If the family is planning to adopt a child from a different culture or race than their own, a specially designed questionnaire is completed by the applicants. This is designed to help the family consider the realities of transracial or transnational adoption. The social worker can use their responses for later discussion as needed and will incorporate this additional information into the adoptive family assessment.

In addition to the use of the questionnaire, the social worker arranges for the applicants to meet with other families who have adopted children from the same or a similar country. Both informal and/or structured formats are used to facilitate discussion, exploration and knowledge sharing.

Special Needs TRACK

The third available series of TRACK Workshops is designed to meet the needs of prospective adoptive parents who plan to adopt a child who is school-aged or has a mental, emotional, or physical disability or applicants who wish to adopt a sibling group. During the three sessions (six-hour curriculum and discussion) of the Special Needs TRACK Preparation, the participants will be provided with knowledge and an understanding of what special needs adoption involves, an understanding of the adoptive child's perspective, and a beginning knowledge base for developing further parenting skills.

The three session series includes discussion of topics on the importance of commitment to the success of adoptions; knowledge and understanding of the behaviors and problems seen in special needs adoption; the importance of attachment; development of effective parenting methods and communication; and resources for the child and various support systems for the family.

CLOSED CIRCUIT TELECONFERENCING IN ADOPTION PREPARATION

As a state agency offering adoption services throughout the state from one central office, the Bureau is faced with the problem of delivering services to clients who live as far as three hours from the central location.

Planning the workshops in the evening is found to be an advantage to most families, however, for some families, adding a two or three hour drive to the schedule could be prohibitive. Social workers and/or panelists traveling to outlying locations in the state in an effort to participate in CORE and TRACK Workshops would also be difficult.

Having identified the educational aspects of the preparation and developed a curriculum built around these concepts, and yet hampered by travel time and scheduling, the possibilities of using the state's educational television network's (SCETV) closed-circuit teleconferencing facilities to transmit adoption preparation workshops from a centrally located studio to technical education sites throughout the state were explored.

The first television conference series called Medical Symposium premiered in 1961 and that teleconference has continued uninterrupted for more than 25 years. In 1961, SCETV had one single channel closed-circuit network penetrating 31 sites in 11 counties; within 24 months, the closed-circuit system was expanded to cover all 46 South Carolina counties. Last year, SCETV delivered 465 full motion video conferences and 322 audio conferences and transmitted more than 1,200 higher education classes by video conferences across the state. In 1985, the network initiated the use of Ku-Band. Today, the SCETV closed-circuit system spans the state with four channels, expanding to eight channels in the larger cities. More than 500 sites are linked by (the) network. SCETV has microwave facilities for simultaneous two-way video-conferencing linking five cities and will increase its two-way capacity to 13 cities by 1988. SCETV is the third largest public broadcast producer in the United States and produces programs at studios, with mobile units and multipoint organizational coordination (Nickerson, 1986).

After initial exploration of the possibility of offering the CORE and TRACK adoption preparation series using telecommunications, it was concluded that South Carolina ETV's Teleconference Design Group could provide a service of live closed-circuit teleconferences hosted in a central studio and transmitted to television screens at any of the 19 technical colleges around the state which are equipped to allow immediate "talk-back."

After the initial contractual arrangements between the agency and SCETV were made by the executive director of the Children's Bureau, production activities began. Planning conferences were held with SCETV's teleconference group. The purpose of the conferences included exchange of knowledge of the objectives of the classes for the teleconference crew and for social work staff, and to provide a basic understanding of various production techniques. One of the first tasks was to develop a "script" which is an especially designed device to assist SCETV production to organize each segment of audio and video transmission. It is the agency's responsibility to develop scripts and provide them to the series producer in advance. With directions provided, the director can move smoothly from one screen to another or from one camera to another at prearranged times. A wraparound system with a moderator introducing and ending the presentation and handling live talk-back questions is currently being used.

The session content consists of a variety of creative formats including testimonial profiles, interviews, and combinations of live panelists and remote interviews which were held with various social workers in their offices. These interviews are shown on split screens with voice-overs combined with the live panelists and activities of the moderator. A question and answer period between participants and the panel or guests is a valuable part of the teleconference since it offers instant reactions over long distances.

The SCETV Teleconference Design Group report that huge savings accompany the teleconference for any state agency or public service group with a message to convey. Money is saved by eliminating most travel costs. Time is saved because participants spend fewer hours away from work and less time is spent planning small group meetings. Energy is saved since any participant in the state only has to travel to the nearest technical center to take part in the program. For example, one social worker in the central studio presented the workshops needed to prepare 80 families. The threefold savings of money, time and energy cannot be ignored, especially in these days of diminishing resources. For example, one social worker in the TV broadcast station can prepare an unlimited number of clients unlike the limited number of clients who can be prepared in a face-to-face, live group process. However, the technical college sites do need volunteer monitors to sign-in clients, collect fees and questionnaires, and make observations about any unusual behaviors. Volunteers are trained and utilized through a contractual arrangement with the South Carolina Council on Adoptable Children (COAC), a child advocacy and adoptive parent support group affiliated with the North America Council on Adoptable Children. Dorothy V. Harris, ACSW, past President of the National Association of Social Workers believes that volunteers, with appropriate training and supervision can function effectively in most settings. We have found this to be true of the volunteer monitors who help with the teleconference preparation of prospective adoptive parents.

Effectiveness is added to efficiency for more productive teleconference broadcasting. Ideas can be presented in interesting ways. Presentations can be enhanced by the use of the following elements: slides, experts presenting live or on video tape, music, printed handouts, artwork, film clips, informal discussion, professional moderators, and panel input to name a few.

An average of 43 individual clients viewed three teleconferences which utilized five sites each time, including the base transmission site in which a monitor was utilized. The clients were asked for written evaluative feedback about the usefulness of the presentations, the quality of the presentations, and the comfort of the facility where they viewed the presentations. Ratings by all but a few were high in all three areas. The few who did not feel the presentations were helpful either did not believe any involvement with the Agency was necessary or had been prepared individually for a previous adoption and thought the presentations to be too simplistic or repetitious. The staff has been far more critical, especially of the more technical production aspects of the teleconferences than have the clients. The staff seems more concerned than the client with such things as the loss of a worker-client relationship because teleconferencing is perceived as a more impersonal presentation of basic educational information. Staff and clients, however, have ample opportunities to develop individual and group relationships later during the specialized "tracks" and home visits. The introduction of the teleconference does contribute to a set of technological complications and problems related to the preparation and taping of the various segments, the scheduling of sites and mechanical as well as electronic malfunctions. These have been overcome through increased cooperative efforts between Bureau, SCETV staff, and COAC volunteers.

The staff at the Bureau conclude that a teleconference is a way to move ideas instead of people, an alternative to the traditional meeting, a money-saving concept, a statewide gathering of people, and an instant sharing of information.

SUMMARY

The Children's Bureau of South Carolina, a centrally located adoption agency serving citizens statewide, recently began utilizing SCETV teleconferencing facilities to broadcast adoption preparation workshops to various technical college sites throughout the state. Before the teleconferencing technology could be utilized, traditional group adoption preparation was reexamined and reformatted into modular units which focused on the educational aspects of preparation. While the production of teleconferencing is definitely "high tech," it is not Hollywood. It is business television. Many advantages to utilizing teleconferencing for the preparation of prospective adoptive parents have been identified. Larger numbers of clients can be served simultaneously. Flexibility in the manner in which the programs can be developed are also distinct advantages. Furthermore, teleconferences are interactive, allowing clients to participate through asking questions throughout the program.

Everything considered, the Agency staff believes that the use of teleconferences in adoption preparation is a useful and worthwhile innovation. The advantages seem to far outweigh the problems and disadvantages. One client captured the sentiments of many when they added the following comment to their evaluation of the teleconference presentation:

> Thank you for preparing me for adoption. I have been enlightened and made aware of a lot of pros and cons to adoption— but the pros were much, much greater. Thank you again!

REFERENCES

Benet, M.K. (1976). *The politics of adoption* (p. 24). New York: Free Press.
Brooks, L.M. & Brooks, E.C. (1939). *Adventuring in adoption* (p. 94). Chapel Hill: The University of North Carolina Press.
Children's Home Society of California, I'm seventeen, I'm pregnant . . . and I don't know what to do (film).
Drake, C., The grafted tree (presentation).

Fink, A. (1949). The field of social work (pp. 18-19). New York: Henry Holt and Company, Inc.

Harris, D.V. (1986). Level of professionalism: An interview with Dorothy V. Harris. *Protecting Children*, *3*, 13.

Nickerson, K. (1986). South Carolina educational television care study. *The Business Communication Magazine*, *5*(3), 22-23.

Index

Printed and bound by CPI Group (UK) Ltd, Croydon, CR0 4YY

17/10/2024

01775662-0001